"Sis",

With love from

Clare

xx

HOPE

Clare Shvili

MINERVA PRESS
ATLANTA LONDON SYDNEY

HOPE

ISBN 0 75410 701 9

First Published 1999 by
MINERVA PRESS
315–317 Regent Street
London W1 7YB

Printed in Great Britain for Minerva Press

HOPE

Dedicated to my mother-in-law, Rachel,
who died from breast cancer in 1996 at the age of sixty-six.

With thanks to all my ladies and their families, also special thanks to my family, Natalie Tidbury and Natalie and Andy Whitehall. I would also like to thank my oncologist, Dr John Scoble, Rabbi Jonathan Romain, all the girls at Breakthrough Breast Cancer and Liz McPherson for their help with my research.

About the Author

I am thirty-eight years old. I've had cancer twice: a breast cancer back in 1993 and a secondary in 1997. Apart from time off for operations, I continued to work throughout, even during the radiotherapy, and in 1994 completed a two-year course converting to Judaism, my husband Giyora's religion. In 1996 I gave birth to our son Nile. How lucky we are!

But, of course, realistically, I know that there is nobody in the world who can tell me how long I've got left on this earth. But I feel good, and to me that's what's most important.

I remember that when I realised cancer was a possibility for me, the first thing I did was rush out and buy a book about somebody's breast cancer experience. That book became my handbook, and I'm sure that all of my ladies had their own handbooks!

This year marks the sixth year from my original diagnosis, so this book seems a most appropriate way in which to celebrate. I am realistic, but optimistic.

Foreword

One in twelve women in Britain will develop breast cancer during their lives, one in ten in Northern Ireland. Fifteen thousand women die each year from breast cancer here in the UK. We have one of the worst mortality rates from the disease in the whole of Europe. Frightening, isn't it?

But for a lot of women the prospects can be good. With early detection and the right treatment, things can look quite different.

This is a collection of stories about survival. These women have opened their hearts and minds for you, the reader. They want to let you know that there is light at the end of the tunnel.

So, read on… I hope you are able to identify with one of them, maybe in age or personality, or just where they come from. Most of all, I hope this book will give strength and courage to anyone facing breast cancer to fight the illness and give hope for the future.

Preface

It is a sad fact that at some point in everyone's life he or she will know someone who has had breast cancer. But by the same token, as time goes on we will all know someone who has survived the disease, and knowing that is tremendously important.

We live in an age where the medical advances are incredible, and I hope that in the next decade or two a cure will have been found for all cancers, and if not a cure then a breakthrough in prevention.

Cancer can be a difficult disease to treat because it is chronic. Although we hear the doctors say there's a 90–95 % chance of beating breast cancer if it is caught in the early stages, what proof do they have that a specific breast cancer is in its early stages? The answer is that they might have indicators, they might have past experiences to go by, and they even have statistics, but none of these can be applied to that remaining 5–10 % of doubt.

One of the most important things is to be aware of breast cancer and its early warning signs. Sometimes there aren't even any of these to make us ask a question, so knowing how to check ourselves is equally important. If we can't do that, we must get the right medical person to do it instead.

By nature, the English are a polite, conservative lot. Very often we're afraid to ask a doctor something that is really worrying us, and when we get told 'It's nothing to worry about' we go home, accept what the doctor has said and then start worrying about it again! True, isn't it? I think we have to learn to take responsibility for our own bodies and take control over decisions to help improve our health.

I know for some people this can be difficult, as not everyone is as outspoken as I am. But reading, knowing and understanding about breast cancer can help the more reserved person get a perspective on the disease…

The problems with breast cancer are many and varied: the fear, the waiting, the not knowing, the surgery, the treatment. So doesn't it make sense to arm ourselves for the battle ahead?

Let's go through all these things, one by one… Fear is a perfectly natural human reaction to the thought that you might have cancer or to being told that you've got cancer. But, in my opinion, without fear there would possibly be no desire to fight the illness. There might be no adrenaline flowing.

The waiting, well, yes, I would have to say this is a difficult stage. But maybe it is a time when you can get yourself straight and organised and be well prepared and ready for what may lie ahead. Reading, talking, finding out about what you need to know – this is the time to be doing these things. However, I offer you a word of warning: unless you truly want to, don't read in-depth medical books. These really can be quite frightening unless you have a medical background.

I wonder how many people prefer not to know what is wrong with them, thinking that it will go away. But I can assure you that however painful it is to find out you have cancer, it is better to know, because once you know, you can do something about it. Ignoring it can only make things worse. Having cancer is all about learning to cope and live with it, just like a bereavement. The difference is that you can do something about the cancer.

The patient can benefit from taking an active role in decisions about his or her surgery and treatment, and although I would never advise anyone to go against specific medical advice, if you're not sure, you are entitled to a second opinion. Also, I think doctors are only too willing to answer your questions. These days, we are seeing more dedicated breast cancer centres being set up, which are able to offer complementary therapies, counselling and support groups.

I think we also have to be careful that we don't knock the medical profession too much. We're all bound to have read about a blunder here or there, but even though they are the professionals, they are also human and have their limitations. It is worth finding a consultant (if possible) who has a particularly keen interest in breast surgery. You must remember that someone like this will do that kind of work because he/she enjoys it and the chances are that he/she is particularly good in this field of work.

This book has been designed to help other women (and men) who are diagnosed with breast cancer so that they do not feel so isolated with their worries and emotions. Maybe it will also help their families, who usually suffer in silence and who are sometimes forgotten by the rest of society.

My last word is about positive thinking and having hope. I was talking to someone recently who was telling me about a woman who had originally been diagnosed with breast cancer five years ago. She had since had various secondaries, and although her ultimate prognosis was not good, she was coping well, living life as normally as she could and was amazing all her doctors! Even my own mother-in-law lived for close on twenty years from her original cancer. Endeavouring to recover, to maintain quality of life, is tremendously important for both the patient and his/her family. We must have hope. Without hope, what is there?

Contents

List of Women Featured		xv
I	Catherine Lord	19
II	Lynda Tavakoli	29
III	Fay Ross	43
IV	Jeanette Sharp	51
V	Viviane Morris	63
VI	Judith James	75
VII	Lynne Middleton	83
VIII	Linda Jacoby	91
IX	Jo Evans	103
X	Jean Hurd	115
XI	Julia Wolfe	125
XII	Doreen Hinder	133
XIII	Sylvia Richards-Jones, MBE	141
Advisory Services		150

List of Women Featured

Catherine Lord	Lives in Cannock Wood, Staffordshire with her husband. She was in her late fifties when the cancer was diagnosed. Her treatment included a mastectomy and she has just finished taking Tamoxifen after five years.
Lynda Tavakoli	Lives in Anahilt, Northern Ireland with her husband and their two children. She was diagnosed with breast cancer in 1993 at the age of thirty-seven. She had surgery and radiotherapy. A year later she had a second malignant lump in the axilla region which was removed and she was then given chemotherapy. She also takes Tamoxifen.
Fay Ross	Lives in Wilton Dean, Hawick with her husband. She was diagnosed with breast cancer in September 1995, when she was in her early forties. She underwent a lumpectomy followed by radiotherapy.

Jeanette Sharp — Lives in Little Haywood, Staffordshire with her husband and young son. She was diagnosed in 1993 when she was in her mid-thirties. She had surgery followed by radiotherapy. In 1997, she gave birth to her little boy.

Viviane Morris — Lives in North London with her husband and two daughters. Had her first breast cancer in 1992 at the age of thirty-six, for which she had a partial mastectomy followed by radiotherapy. In 1997 she had a second breast cancer. Another partial mastectomy and radiotherapy followed.

Judith James — Lives in Hawarden, Flintshire with her husband and has two grown-up sons. She was diagnosed with breast cancer in 1993 at the age of forty-nine. She had a mastectomy and now takes Tamoxifen.

Lynne Middleton — Lives in Cults, Aberdeen with her husband and two children. She was diagnosed in 1997 at the age of forty-two. She had surgery, chemotherapy and radiotherapy. Now she is on Tamoxifen.

Linda Jacoby	Lives in Maidenhead, Berkshire with her husband and two teenage daughters. Her breast cancer was diagnosed in 1995 when she was forty-two. She had surgery followed by radiotherapy and is now taking Tamoxifen.
Jo Evans	Lives with her boyfriend in Liverpool. She was diagnosed with breast cancer in 1997 when she was in her mid-twenties. She had surgery followed by radiotherapy and has been on Tamoxifen ever since.
Jean Hurd	Lives near to Cheadle, Cheshire. She is widowed and has two grown-up daughters and two grandchildren. She was diagnosed with breast cancer in 1993 when she was in her fifties. She had surgery and radiotherapy and was prescribed Tamoxifen.
Julia Wolfe	Lives in London with her husband and two young children. She had breast cancer in 1995 when she was in her mid-thirties. She had surgery, chemotherapy and radiotherapy, and was given Tamoxifen.

Doreen Hinder — Lives in Stanwix, Carlisle with her husband. Her breast cancer was diagnosed in 1996 while in her fifties. She underwent a mastectomy and was put on Tamoxifen. She has since had reconstructive surgery.

Sylvia Richards-Jones MBE — Lives in Brymbo, Wrexham with her husband. They have two grown-up children and two grandchildren. She was diagnosed in 1996 when in her late fifties. After having a mastectomy, she was put on Tamoxifen.

Chapter I
Catherine Lord

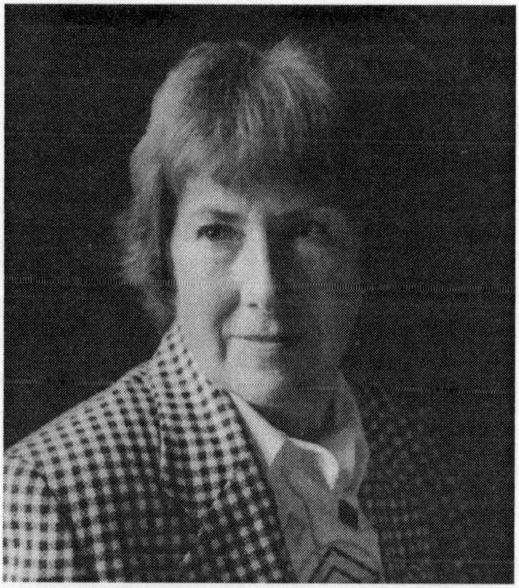

Photo by Clare Shvili, 1998

Catherine Lord lives in Cannock Wood, Staffordshire with her husband. She was in her late fifties when the cancer was diagnosed. Her treatment included a mastectomy and she has just finished taking Tamoxifen after five years.

Catherine's Story

It was back in January 1998 that I rang Catherine to arrange a meeting. The dulcet tones of a Scotswoman took me by surprise. I was expecting a broad Rugeley accent which couldn't be much more different than a Scottish one.

We arranged to meet at her golf club which is right in the heart of Cannock Chase. It was a bitterly cold day but the sun shone in great hues through the tall bare trees that lined the road.

I got lost. In fact, I was terribly lost and for a while I seemed to be driving round in circles (which is easy to do on Cannock Chase). Eventually I found a sign for the golf club and followed a very grand driveway up to the clubhouse. It was only then that I started to wonder what she'd look like: I reckoned tall, possibly well built.

As I drove into the car park, I suddenly felt incredibly unimportant. I was after all no more than a medically retired housewife playing the role of an up-and-coming author looking for Pulitzer victory! I didn't have a tape recorder or a briefcase, not even a mobile phone, you know, just in case the office wanted me (I don't think so!). But I did have a notepad and pen. What else would I need?

As I walked to the front door of the clubhouse, the cold winter air braced me and my confidence returned as quickly as a shower first thing in the morning wakes you up. Suddenly I wondered how I would recognise her amongst a crowd of strangers. Would she still be there? I was so late that she could have got fed up and gone home.

My internal questions were brought to an abrupt halt. As I entered the hallway, a woman emerged from a side room and asked if I was looking for Catherine. I was a bit taken aback. She must have been watching for my arrival. I hardly had time to reply before she led me up the staircase and into a big social room which was completely empty apart from three chaps playing on the snooker tables.

'This way,' she said. I followed obediently behind and then, almost out of nowhere, there she was!

'This is Catherine,' she said and disappeared quietly. The sun was pouring into the room from behind her and it was hard to see her face properly. Catherine stood up and, holding out her hand, walked towards me. I remember that beam she gave me, how welcoming, how reassuring. I realised at that point that I didn't need any recorder or posey phone. She was happy just to meet *me*!

We chatted for a while and then ordered a drink and some lunch. We found a table in the corner out of the sunlight. Now I had the chance to look at her properly and I had to laugh to myself as all my preconceptions about her appearance were completely wrong. She was small with a slight frame and dark shiny hair, and I thought how attractive she was for a woman in her sixties.

She looked so healthy it was hard to believe that she'd had cancer, but she had, five years before. It was amazing!

I felt a bit tongue-tied. This was the first one. I stammered my way through some questions at the same time as I tackled a tuna toastie. But then, to my relief, she took over and I just leant back and listened.

She had grown up on the Isle of Skye, one of eight children. It sounded like an idyllic childhood, living in a beautiful place, surrounded by a doting family. But the ideals of this childhood seem to have disappeared by adulthood. As she continued with her story, I became paralysed with disbelief.

The eldest sister had died from leukaemia at the age of forty. This was unquestionably distressing and untimely, but there was more to come. A second sister had died several years before, this time from breast cancer. Then Catherine's youngest sister died, also from breast cancer, just before Catherine got her own diagnosis. Her beautiful eyes welled up with tears as she told me how each one in turn had battled and coped with their burden.

She also told me that her brother's son had died from skin cancer and that she also had a sister-in-law with breast cancer. How could one family have so much cancer?

'How did you cope with all this?' I asked.

'Well you just get on with it,' came the reply!

After a while, I realised it was this kind of attitude that had preserved this lass. I asked if she minded talking in so much detail about the rest of her family but the answer was a very positive 'No'. She was obviously full of love and admiration for all these people. Incredibly, her mother lived to ninety-two years of age, but her father had unfortunately died in 1942 after an operation for ulcers.

After hearing all this, I realised that there was no question about her own cancer being the result of a genetic fault.

'So how did it all start?' I continued.

'I went for a check-up when my third sister was going through her treatment. I felt I owed it to myself, just in case. The GP told me that I was on a waiting list for a mammogram anyway, so I went away and waited. Then, a short while after this, I noticed a very slight bloody discharge from one breast. With the knowledge I had, I knew this could be a clinical sign of breast cancer so I went straight back to the GP. He knew about my family history and was very good in that he wasted no time in arranging for a mammogram to be done.'

She continued. 'We got the result of the mammogram back and it was clear! But there was a nagging doubt at the back of my mind and I just felt it needed to be looked at further. My GP asked for the plates to be re-examined and again they came back clear.'

'So what happened next?' I asked.

'He sent me to see the consultant at hospital.'

I wondered what on earth was going through her mind at this point.

Catherine looked at me thoughtfully and said, 'I just wanted it to be thoroughly examined, just in case there was something.' Even though I didn't know her at this point, I could well imagine her determination. There had to be no messing about. Breast cancer, if it was, only meant one thing to her – *death*.

The consultant suggested a small operation to remove a breast duct to look out for any changes. She had a duct removed on 24th January.

'My husband Stephen came with me to get the results a week later. Although I had suspected that all was not well, it was still a real blow when he told us that he had found cancerous cells. I remember turning to my husband and saying "Do you think I can handle this?" "Of course you can," he replied reassuringly. I thought of my nephew and how well he was coping at the time with the knowledge that he had less than six years to live.

'At the time, the consultant did think that I should have a double mastectomy, in view of the family history. But I had some time to think about it, and the decision was to be mine. I went off to have yet another mammogram and saw the breast care nurse and the doctor in the breast care unit. I then saw the oncologist and it was after seeing him that I made the decision to have just the one breast removed.'

So the following Monday, Catherine went into hospital again. It was late February. She had the operation on the Tuesday, was back home on the Sunday and, as she put it, was 'chipping balls' in her kitchen on the Monday.

There is no doubt that she was lucky. Unlike other cases, she had had no lump but had pushed for the investigations, and after the results of the mastectomy came back, they proved she had been right to do so because every duct had been affected.

I wondered at this point how her husband was coping. 'There was no question about it,' she continued. 'He was very supportive throughout. We survived my cancer!'

'I was advised to lay off the golf for three months.' She looked at me and laughed as she said this. 'Well of course I didn't!' Now why didn't that come as any surprise?

Eight months later she became vice-captain of the ladies' section at her golf club. This is her passion – swinging an iron, getting a birdie!

In December 1994 she became captain of the ladies. She saw here an opportunity to use her position to raise some money. She felt that she wanted to be able to give something back to the people who had helped her.

First of all, Catherine had to get permission from the golf club's Board of Managers. Once that was achieved she got stuck in straight away. She arranged and organised lots of events, including a carol concert, coffee mornings, golf competitions and a gala evening held at the club. The fund-raising was endless, her motivation flawless.

She paused for a second as she relayed all this information. Then she continued. 'You know, one day I played a hole of golf at each of forty different golf clubs to raise money!'

For a moment I sat back and looked at this woman. Had she really once had cancer? It was hard to believe. There was no need to ask her what had got her through. It was her fighting spirit, her zest for life.

Amazingly, she finally raised a grand total of eleven thousand pounds which was split equally between the breast care unit at Stafford and St Giles Hospice in Whittington, near Lichfield.

She says that she hopes she's a better and more sympathetic person as a result of her brush with death. Each day is very special to her and she really appreciates each morning when she wakes up and feels so alive and well.

More than six years down the line and now in her early sixties, Catherine remains in remission.

Catherine's Friend's Thoughts

Thoughts from the time when Catherine had cancer:
What are we feeling when in the confines of our home?
What are the hurdles we have to face?
What does the future hold?
Decisions are not just a personal thing; there are others to consider…
They may be hurting just as much.
Empathy is what is needed, not sympathy!
A positive attitude from family and friends.
Valued judgements from the medics.
Others have been through already and have survived.
Don't look back, just forward to what you want…

Chapter II
Lynda Tavakoli

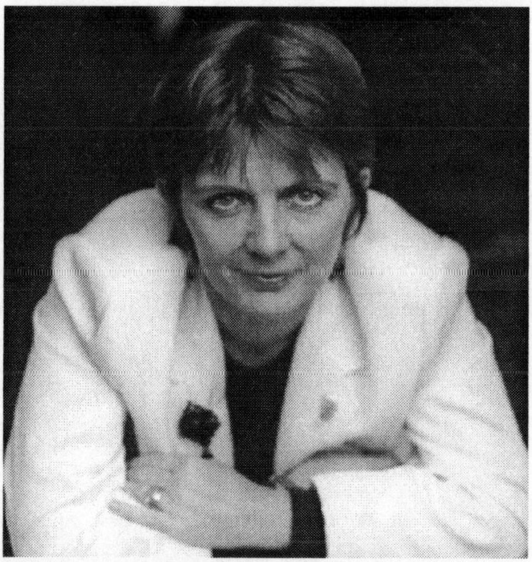

Photo by Clare Shvili, 1998

Lynda Tavakoli lives in Anahilt, Northern Ireland with her husband and their two children. She was diagnosed with breast cancer in 1993 at the age of thirty-seven. She had surgery and radiotherapy. A year later she had a second malignant lump in the axilla region which was removed and she was then given chemotherapy. She also takes Tamoxifen.

Lynda's Story

Sincere, warm, caring – that's Lynda. Never liking to ask others for help but always willing to give herself. Is this kind of personality destined to have breast cancer, I wonder? In reality, we don't know. It is for you the reader to look deep between the lines and decide.

I first received a letter from Lynda at the beginning of the year. There were a lot of things that interested me about this Irish lass so I wrote back and asked her to send me her story. She did, all thirty-three pages of it! It was a lovely piece of writing, but how could I possibly write that much in one chapter? For that reason alone you are reading the edited version.

Lynda was born 2nd May, 1955 in Portadown, Northern Ireland. She was the youngest of three children. From what she has told me, I can only imagine that hers was a cosy Irish childhood, with her mum (whom she refers to as Mummy) being at home full-time to look after them all, while her Dad was a manager at a ready-mix concrete company.

I would say that her family was very close, probably still is, although they are spread out all over the country.

She ended up teaching music at a secondary school in Armagh, but in 1980 when she was twenty-five decided to head off to the States for some excitement. Whether she found it or not I do not know, but she did meet and marry her husband Siamak there, and shortly after they returned to Britain, to a small village just outside Cardiff.

Lynda started to teach special needs children, which was her main interest. In 1987 their daughter Farah was born. Not long after they moved to Sheffield with Siamak's job and Ben was born in 1988. This was not the last move. In 1992 Siamak got a promotion which involved him moving to Belfast. So although Lynda stayed in Sheffield for a time after (in order to sell the house), eventually it brought her full circle and back to her roots.

Then, in the autumn of 1992, her ordeal started. This is what she wrote:

> The lump came first, I guess. But not mine. My Aunt Lily had been diagnosed with breast cancer and was about to have a complete mastectomy. It made me think more about the disease and I decided to examine my own breasts. That's when I found my lump.
>
> My reaction was one of curiosity. How could a lump suddenly appear out of nowhere? I instinctively knew what it was – there was no question. The next day I bought a book about cancer, not out of any morbid sense of death but purely for practical reasons to help me deal with the situation.
>
> The following weekend Siamak was back in Sheffield on one of his fortnightly visits from Belfast. I got him to feel the lump. He estimated it was about a quarter of an inch. That's me exaggerating, I thought, as I had guessed it to be about three quarters of an inch.
>
> On the Monday, when Siamak had returned to Belfast, I went to my GP. The doctor agreed that there was definitely a lump. Four weeks later I was on my way to hospital to see the consultant. I wasn't filled with dread, just uncertainty. After seeing him, I was sent for a mammogram and ultrasound scan. And so the waiting began. The results arrived a few days before Christmas. Everything appeared normal. It made Christmas a lot easier that year.
>
> At the beginning of the New Year I went back to the hospital for a routine check-up. This time I saw the consultant's senior houseman. He asked if I'd noticed any increase in the size of the lump. Well, I

wasn't sure, but I said I thought it was slightly bigger. After reading my notes he'd obviously decided what the next course of action would be. And so he proceeded to do a Fine Needle Aspiration, where some fluid is drawn off for examination. The results would take three weeks to come back, but after making another appointment I left having made the decision to wait for these results before anything else was done.

However, Siamak's reaction was very different. He thought the lump should be removed whatever, and with this resting heavily on my mind, I decided to phone the consultant's secretary for an appointment to go into hospital and have the lump out. Two weeks later it was done. The road to Hassleville had begun.

It was approximately two weeks before the hospital sent word for me to get the results of the biopsy. Two weeks can be a long time in many ways but I certainly didn't spend it worrying and fretting about the outcome. Many people have said to me, since my illness, that everything must have been dreadfully difficult with Siamak away most of the time. In a perverse sort of way, it actually made things easier!

I was so busy with the children that there simply wasn't time to think too deeply. When you've got to deal with things yourself, you just do. I don't mean in an isolated way, but more that you feed on the support of people around you and just get on with it. The support was there if I needed it, but it was never forced on me. I wasn't scared of what was happening to me; in fact what did happen was that I became hungry for information and soon I knew everything there was available to know about breast cancer, just in case the axe did fall.

Practically all my friends in Dronfield had young children and led very busy lives themselves. One friend was a man called Bryan who was in fact a kind of house-husband and whose son went to the same school as Farah. He and his wife Kate had been very kind to me during Siamak's absence and on the day I was due to get the result, Bryan offered to drive me to hospital and wait around to take me home afterwards.

We arrived at the hospital and made our way to the breast clinic. It was packed with people and it was difficult to find a couple of seats. I reported to reception and sat down next to Bryan. As we waited, patients were constantly disappearing into the endless rooms along the corridor and reappearing again at various intervals.

Suddenly a nurse appeared and made a muffled attempt at pronouncing my name. With a surname like Tavakoli, it always causes problems! I gathered my belongings and followed her into one of the rooms. There was a bed in it and an adjoining door leading to the room next door. I knew the procedure – top half of clothes off and onto the bed.

After a while an Asian doctor came in. There was no nurse with him and he asked me to lie down while he examined the site of the operation. And then, just like that, he told me that I had a malignant tumour which required further surgery. My mind was racing. Suddenly I couldn't think straight and I couldn't quite sort out whether 'malignant' meant good or bad! 'Does that mean I have cancer?' I stuttered.

It obviously did. Somehow I managed to get my clothes on and was called into the next room to speak with the doctor. He looked at me and asked if I had any questions. *Any questions?* Now there was an understatement if ever there was! I think I must have been in a state of shock for I had to ask everything about three times and even then I wasn't quite sure what he was telling me. Gradually it sank in and I started to realise that I was going to have some or all of my breast removed and possibly undergo further treatment afterwards. When we'd eventually sorted things out I walked out of the room in a bit of a daze.

Bryan patently took the news a lot worse than I did, which under the circumstances was not surprising. He'd given up his afternoon to run me to the hospital and home again probably never suspecting for one moment that all this was going to happen.

Before we were able to leave, I was sent to have a chest x-ray and a blood test. Eventually it was all over and we left. On the way back, Bryan and I hardly knew what to say to each other.

We picked the kids up and then Bryan drove us back home. As it was winter, it was already dark outside. We arrived back home to find it in complete darkness. Bryan asked if I wanted him to come in and talk for a while but I said no. He had his own family waiting for him and, to be honest, I just wanted to be on my own with the kids. I knew that the night ahead of me was going to be tough.

Everyone who phoned me that evening was as shocked as the last one and that included my mum. But although shocked, she remained pretty calm and practical about it all. After all, what can a person say? The worst they can do is react with horror and cry hysterically, but I'm not from that sort of family, and, good or not, it has stood me in good stead.

After talking with Mum I set about getting the children ready for bed. Just as I was putting them down the phone went again and I knew it had to be Siamak. There is no tactful way of telling someone you have cancer so I simply, in a very matter-of-fact way, related all the events of the day. It must have been terribly difficult for him to take it all in and the fact that the great Irish Sea lay between us didn't help.

I suppose he must have felt that he should have been there with me. My overriding feeling was one of gratitude that it had been he who had persuaded me to have the lump removed in the first place. I shudder to think what would have been if it had been left up to me.

It was obvious that my surgery would have to be fairly immediate and I was booked in for a week later. Siamak had to get time off work to stay at home and look after the kids. On 23rd February I went in for the operation. Within the first few hours I was visited by my allocated nurse, a student nurse, an anaesthetist, the breast care nurse and most importantly by the consultant. He explained the procedure. Technically he was going to perform a wide excision lumpectomy with axillary node clearance.

And so, there I was again, being wheeled through the corridors down to the theatre. The next thing I remember was waking up already back on the ward and in real pain. A shot of morphine sorted that out.

The following day the consultant paid me another visit and said that the surgery had gone well. Now all I had to do was wait for two days until the results came through. It seemed like a very long wait but eventually the day came.

It was a Thursday and Siamak had come to visit me while the kids were at school. Suddenly out of the blue the consultant appeared. He had come up especially with my results and was delighted to tell me that the lymph nodes were clear. The relief was immense. Life was not so bleak after all and the future seemed almost bright. I had, by this time, had the bandages removed and was pleased with the result of the surgery. The cut was about one and a half inches long but very neat. There was another smaller cut higher in my armpit where the lymph nodes had been removed. On Thursday evening I returned home and in many ways I was relieved to get out of hospital.

Very shortly after coming out of hospital, my radiotherapy began. It would go on for six weeks. Each morning the routine was the same. I would check in at the reception desk, wait to be called, find a cubicle and change into a gown, and then wait to be called in for the actual treatment. The whole thing took no longer than ten minutes and was completely painless. The only change to this routine occurred during the sixth week when a different machine was used and I was marked out differently for the treatment.

Having finished my course of radiotherapy I had one final appointment to see the doctor. A while before I'd had a bone scan and he now told me that the result of the scan was fine and that he felt that overall my prognosis was very good. Our house move was now imminent and he was going to forward all my notes to Belvoir Park Hospital in Northern Ireland. In fact, we moved house the following week so there was very little time to think of anything but getting packed up and leaving.

In Ireland, I would continue to be seen every three months until further notice. The first appointment in the oncology department went well and it was agreed that everything that could be done had been done. I went home to start living a normal life again and put my ordeal behind me.

Life went on and our first Christmas in Northern Ireland loomed ahead. A couple of weeks before the festivities I did one of my regular breast checks, feeling deep into the armpit as I had been told to do. I could hardly believe it but there it was – another lump!

My next appointment at the oncology clinic was in the new year, on Farah's birthday in fact, the fourth of January. I had made the decision not to tell Siamak or my parents about this new lump as it would serve little purpose except to worry them half to death and spoil Christmas for everyone.

So here I was again, the scenario was familiar. I arrived at the clinic and saw the doctor who examined me and asked about my general health. I waited until after he'd finished examining me before I mentioned this new lump because he obviously hadn't felt it himself. Eventually he detected it and concluded that it needed to be removed in order, to make a diagnosis. Well, I knew that!

Siamak took the news well under the circumstances and remained very calm. Meanwhile, I started to read everything I could get my hands on that could tell me more about my condition. The reality of what might lie ahead suddenly struck me and I could only envisage even more disruption for the family ahead.

There was then only a short time to wait before going into the Belfast City Hospital and I was on a special breast care ward. Soon I was back on the operating table yet again.

I cannot remember what time I arrived back on the ward. I vaguely remember waking up in the recovery room at one stage but must have fallen asleep again. I was in no pain when I finally came round. In fact, I felt fine in myself and by early evening I was sitting up in bed. At about nine o'clock I went to phone Siamak. I knew he'd be at home with the kids because we'd agreed it would be pointless visiting me that evening.

The next day on the ward there was a feeling of apprehension. Everyone was aware that when the doctors did their rounds that evening it was 'results' time. The day wore on and eventually there was a great buzz on the ward that 'they' had arrived. I almost fell into a state of panic at that point for there was still no sign of Siamak, but then, just as the doctors were entering the ward, the lift doors opened and there he was.

Soon the curtains were being pulled round my bed and the doctor walked through. His face told the story. With my history it shouldn't have come as a shock but all the same it was a real blow.

He said the lump they had taken from the axilla had contained cancer cells which meant there had been spread from the primary site. It was the first time that I allowed myself to cry. When I regained my composure it was time to talk about the practicalities of the situation. An oncologist was to see me either later that evening or the next morning. And then the doctor moved on. After Siamak left, I sat and tried to work out where to go from here.

Once I'd returned home, I prepared myself for the forthcoming appointment with the oncologist. I started reading again, although Siamak thought I was reading too much. But it was my way of coping.

The day arrived and Siamak went with me. As I had done all my 'research' beforehand, I was well aware of the treatment that would be on offer. It was decided that I would have eight sessions of chemo which would be spaced three weeks apart in order to allow my body to recover in between sessions. Each time I went I would have my blood counts checked as they are all affected by the drugs.

All in all, I have to say that my chemotherapy treatment was pretty straight forward and not nearly as horrific as some of the stories I'd heard about, but then again not everyone reacts in the same way.

Finally, when the chemo was at an end, I went back to the hospital to have my ovaries irradiated. I headed straight into an early menopause and all that it brings with it. The only remaining medication for me to take was Tamoxifen, which I started almost immediately after the chemo and have been taking a 20 mg daily dose ever since.

But my main reason for writing this is not because I'm any kind of special person but so that I can tell someone else that I've weathered the storm and may even be a better person for it. My future is by no means certain, but then whose is?

With a disease like breast cancer the only way forward is positive thinking and I'm quite sure I've got enough of that to take me anywhere I want to go!

Lynda's Sister Jean's Story

When Lynda's cancer was first diagnosed I have to say I was surprised at how she reacted. She told me that when she examined herself she just knew that she'd find something. My own initial reaction was one of shock. But then straight away the practical side kicked in. Pity really does no good in this sort of situation. I think when something like this happens, you've got to be real about it and approach it from the point of view of, 'This is it. What can I do about it?'

I tried to help when I could. And I've never been afraid to talk about it. I think it helps to talk.

I went along to Lynda's support group. When you see the empty chairs and you know they're empty for the wrong reason, that's very moving. But the sense of camaraderie within the group is really inspiring and really positive.

Since Lynda was diagnosed I've been taking part in trials at Heath Hospital in Cardiff to study the possibility of genetic links. They've assessed my risk factor, which as it turns out isn't significantly higher. I don't know how I would react if I was told that I had cancer. But I would like to think that I would cope in the way Lynda has.

The overriding thing in all of this is how much I admire what Lynda has done. She's turned something very rotten into something positive. I have nothing but admiration for her motivation and inspiration.

When something as major as this comes along, you don't know how you'll deal with it. But I think when it comes really close, you do find the strength to cope with what's sitting on your shoulder.

Early detection is so important. I teach at a girls' school and we held a special assembly during Breast Cancer Awareness Month last year to talk to the girls about the disease. I think it's vitally important to raise awareness. You don't want to scare people but you do want to put across the idea that it is something to be careful about.

I do think about the disease but don't spend nights agonising about it. When you're really happy and you're almost at that point where you want to stop the world and make everything stand still, that's when you think about it.

Chapter III
Fay Ross

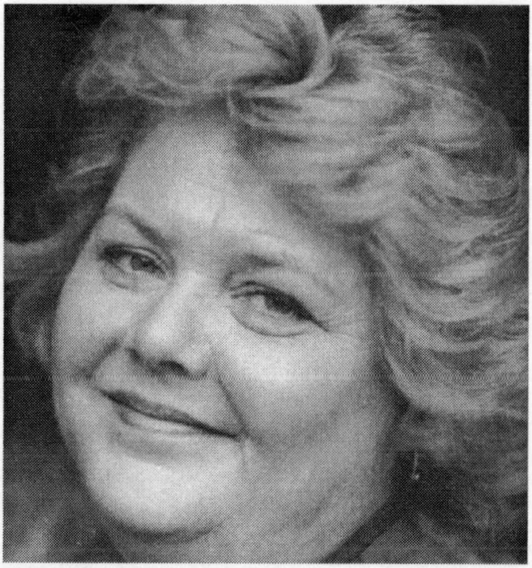

Photo by Clare Shvili, 1998

Fay Ross lives in Wilton Dean, Hawick with her husband. She was diagnosed with breast cancer in September 1995, when she was in her early forties. She underwent a lumpectomy followed by radiotherapy.

Fay's Story

You only have to look at Fay's picture to see what sort of person she is; fun-loving with a real sense of humour. When she first wrote to me, I had to look up 'Hawick' on the map, I'd never heard of it before, but sure enough, there it was in the middle of all those Scottish glens! And of course, as you'd expect, she has an accent to go with it, although not a larger-than-life one – more of a sweet, mischievous one!

Fay was born in Hawick and has in fact never lived anywhere else. It is only a small place with a population of about fifteen thousand. It is mainly known for its beautiful cashmere sweaters: companies such as Pringle of Scotland and Lyle and Scott operate here.

Her mother's first husband was killed in Burma during the war and she married Fay's father, who was a bricklayer, in 1950. Fay was born in 1951 and has three brothers and a sister. Unfortunately, both her parents are now dead. Her mother died suddenly from a heart attack in 1986 and her father from lung cancer in 1990. From the way she wrote, the memory of her father's illness and treatment is obviously still strong in her mind.

She left school without bothering to take any O levels, much to her parents' disgust. She went to work as a dental nurse in one of the local practices and then went on to become the wages clerk for a knitwear company, which she has done for a long time now.

I was looking for a possible reason for her breast cancer. Diet, smoking and contraception were all things that I asked her about.

She says she has always had a battle with her weight and has tried every diet going without much success. She has smoked off and on since she was sixteen, mainly as, what she would call a social smoker, but stopped altogether after her father was diagnosed with lung cancer. On the last point of contraception, she has never taken the pill, and so the question of a trigger factor remains.

In 1988, Fay discovered her first breast lump. She had it removed and it turned out to be benign, although she had never doubted that it was anything else. Then, in 1995, after not feeling well for a while, she went to see a lady doctor who prescribed Hormone Replacement Therapy for Fay. To begin with, she felt uneasy about taking it, partly because of her weight problem and also because of the uncertainty about the possible risks of it increasing the chances of breast cancer. However, after reading the literature she had been given by the doctor and also watching a video, she decided to give it a go.

After about two months, she started to feel like her old self again. In fact she hadn't felt so well for more than two years and was really grateful that the doctor had suggested the HRT. She felt much happier in herself and actually lost a stone in weight. Then she and her husband went on holiday to Turkey; she was obviously in good form!

But eight weeks later, one night when she was examining her breasts she noticed a puckering about the size of a fifty-pence piece. It was fortunate that she had checked herself in front of the wardrobe mirror on this occasion and not in the bath as she normally did.

She phoned the surgery about a week later as the puckering was still there. Her own doctor was very busy, and so she took the first appointment available which was with a female locum, who was very nice and helpful. The doctor referred Fay to see a specialist, which she felt all right about. Besides which, she had been through all this once before. When she went home later and told her husband, she was certain that this time she had breast cancer.

She got an appointment within two weeks and went along to her local cottage hospital to see the consultant. He did a fine needle aspiration in which some cells were drawn off for examination. He was totally honest and said the puckering could be caused by a tumour inside which might have tethered itself to the overlying skin. He told Fay that even if the result of the needle test was normal, he might still want to operate.

Fay asked him to telephone her as soon as he had the results and gave him both her home and work telephone numbers. She had heard about him before from other people and felt confident about his ability. But even as she left this appointment, she was still convinced of the result,

Four days later she still hadn't heard anything so Fay rang her sister-in-law who worked at the GP's surgery. Fay was promised that as soon as the doctor knew the result someone would phone her. In fact it was the consultant himself who rang her at lunchtime. He said that there was something wrong and that he wanted her to go into the local general hospital the following Monday for further tests. Five minutes after she had put the phone down to the consultant, the locum called. She arranged to meet Fay and her husband at home that afternoon.

Fay remembers how kind the doctor was when she arrived. She says that the doctor really listened to what she had to say. After the doctor had left, Fay phoned some of her friends. She felt that they didn't really know what to say to her but assured her that she'd be okay. She wondered afterwards how on earth they could know whether she'd be all right or not, but of course this is a common reply from someone who is neither experienced nor directly involved with such a situation. People simply don't know what else to say!

Amazingly, Fay was never afraid that she might die and was prepared to have her breast removed if necessary. That weekend, she and her husband went to Carlisle on the Saturday morning to buy her some nighties from Marks and Spencer, and in the afternoon they went to the races! They finished off their day with a lovely meal and one can only imagine that they were determined to enjoy themselves before the turmoil began.

On the Monday morning, Fay went into hospital to have a bone scan, a mammogram, a blood test and finally a chest x-ray. She was allowed to go home afterwards, but had to return the following afternoon. This, she says, was the hardest part, waiting and wondering if the cancer had spread. When she returned on the Tuesday she asked to have a private room, which she was granted on the proviso that if there was someone else who needed it, such as a difficult patient, she would have to give it up. To this, her husband quipped that they didn't come any more difficult than Fay!

Her operation was done on the Thursday morning, first thing. A lumpectomy was performed and some glands from the axilla were also removed. The surgery actually helped to even up the size of her breasts as the right one had always been slightly bigger.

All the results were encouraging, and although the tumour was confirmed as being malignant, there was no spread to either the lymph glands or anywhere else. Fay was offered surgery to even up the nipples, but as she said herself, she wouldn't be auditioning for Baywatch and if that was all she had to worry about, then it wasn't much!

But once she was back at home, she became obsessed with reading about breast cancer. She would go from being full of confidence to full of complete despair. She worried about the possibility of having chemotherapy as her father had done, and the effects that this can have.

Once the wound had healed, she had five weeks of radiotherapy at the Western General in Edinburgh. She stayed in a place called Raeburn House from Monday to Friday while she was having the treatment. Whilst she was there, she got out and about and spent an absolute fortune shopping! But this was her way of coping. If she'd have stayed in all the time, surrounded by people who were in a worse state than herself, she thinks she would have crumbled.

She sailed through the treatment, and it was only during the final week that her skin started to take the toll from the radiotherapy, but this was short-lived. The only things she remembers from this time are really quite trivial, such as not being allowed to wash the area of treatment properly or use deodorant.

When she got back home, the tiredness she experienced was the main problem. One minute she could feel fine and then the next minute be completely knackered. Five weeks later she started back at work part-time, gradually building up her hours each week until she was back full-time.

There are some good things that have come out of Fay's cancer experience. Firstly, she thinks that she and her husband are closer than before, and although she says he is a typical Scotsman who would rather die than admit his feelings, she feels that there have been times when it's been harder for him to cope than for her, and this in turn has made them stronger.

She is very open about her illness, especially if she feels she can reassure other people that you can come through it. At the time of writing, Fay is nearly four years down the line and fighting fit!

Fay's Husband's Story

After Fay found the second lump in her breast, I was overwhelmed with fear and anxieties even though the first one had been benign. Waiting for the test results was a strain on us both and then once we had the diagnosis, the worry was whether the disease had spread to anywhere else in her body.

We would only have these answers after the operation. All the discussions we had with the doctors and medical staff were very encouraging, and everyone was very positive for Fay. People showed us nothing but kindness and support.

For me, it was a very difficult time as I was trying to get a new business off the ground at the same time as all this was going on. 1996 was a year that Fay and I would like to forget. However, I do believe that Fay's awareness of the risk of breast cancer saved her life.

If telling Fay's story can help to make more women aware of breast cancer and the need for early detection, then some good will have been done.

Chapter IV
Jeanette Sharp

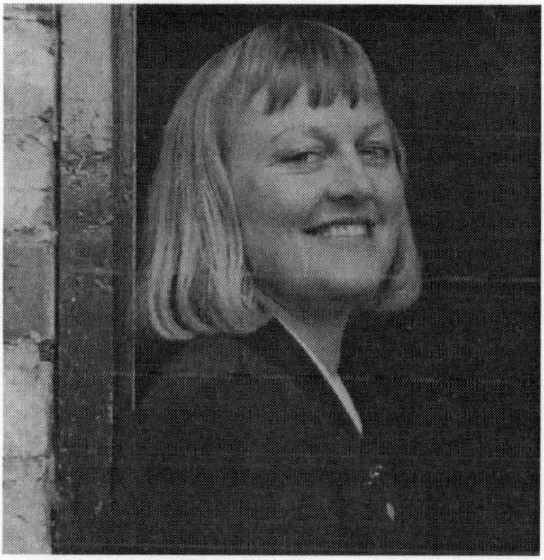

Photo by Clare Shvili, 1998

Jeanette Sharp lives in Little Haywood, Staffordshire with her husband and young son. She was diagnosed in 1993 when she was in her mid-thirties. She had surgery followed by radiotherapy. In 1997, she gave birth to her little boy.

Jeanette's Story

Jeanette and I have a lot in common. Not only do we share the same oncologist, but we're almost the same age and have both had babies after our cancers! So it was for these reasons that it was particularly nice to meet up with her one evening and talk about her story.

Most people I've met who've had breast cancer, physically, don't give you any clues about what they've been through, and Jeanette was no exception.

When she opened the door to me, there was a slim, fit-looking girl welcoming me into her home. There was no need for pleasantries. We knew exactly where the other one was coming from. We chatted for a couple of hours and I met her husband, Kim. Around the room were several photos of her little boy, Christopher, and it was obvious to me that whatever they'd gone through, it was well and truly behind them now.

Being of a similar age to her at the diagnosis stage, I was curious to know what she thought had been the cause of her illness. She believed it had been stress induced. Seven years before her cancer, she had gone through a pretty stressful time in her life and she really felt that this had been the trigger point. I could relate enormously to this, having gone through something similar.

There seemed to be nothing else in her background that could have been contributory. She was born and bred in Nottingham. Her dad, who originated from Scotland, was a miner and her mum took care of Jeanette and her older sister at home. They had a well-balanced diet and there is nothing to suggest that Jeanette was not a normal, healthy girl.

She only moved when she went to do a teacher-training course at the West Midlands College in Walsall. She started teaching in 1979 and ten years later married her husband. They now live close to Cannock Chase in Staffordshire.

When I left her home, we arranged that she would send me her written story. It seemed a lot more sensible than trying to remember everything she had told me. What she wrote was easy to understand and precise. She entitled it: *The Enemy Within.*

The Enemy Within

When I first considered writing about my experiences of breast cancer for this book I was a little reticent. Was it tempting fate or not? Would it make me sound overconfident? How would I feel once I'd produced my contribution if the illness recurred? But, as you put it, Clare, one could go on forever more being fatalistic; it is better to live life to the full as you never know what lies ahead. This sounds like a terrible cliché, but there is a great deal of truth in it.

I decided that if I could become ill – me, the person who had barely had a day's illness in her life – it could happen to anyone, and this was all the more reason for me to make a contribution. This is not intended as a warning to any naturally healthy person with confidence in their health, but it is intended, I hope to act as a source of help or comfort to anyone who, as I did, feels that their body has let them down in some way. Coming to terms with this is, I feel, one of the most difficult aspects of the illness.

Physically, I've always considered myself very fit. I have exercised regularly, eaten a reasonably healthy diet and always believed in my physical and mental strength. To be diagnosed with breast cancer was a devastating blow and even to this day I have difficulty trying to convince myself that there was anything wrong with me. What is more, other people were equally as shocked as I was never ill, and barely ever had time off work with illness. That was something that happened to other people, not me!

1992

It all started with the discovery of a pea-shaped lump in the upper part of my left breast. This moved around when pressed. I was a little concerned but not unduly so, and Kim's feeling was the same. But over the next few weeks, I kept noticing it and eventually Kim suggested that I go to the GP.

It was November when I went for the check. My GP didn't seem particularly concerned and reassured me that at the age of thirty-four, it was unlikely to be anything serious. He thought it might be a fibro-adenoma, which is a lump of fibrous tissue and not normally harmful. However, as a precautionary measure, he sent me for an appointment with the consultant at the hospital.

I went to hospital in the February of 1993. He reiterated what my GP had said, that it was a fibro-adenoma and that it might disappear of its own accord. He asked me to return in April for a check-up.

By April the lump was now plainly visible and seemed closer to the surface of the skin. It didn't appear to be any bigger but I was a bit concerned about the way it was changing. The thought that it might be something serious had not really occurred to me. In a way I suppose that I felt almost invincible; this was just a minor blip in an otherwise spotless health record! If my husband had any reservations at this time, he kept them well hidden. It has only been recently that he has revealed that he had an inkling that something was not right.

So I went back to see the consultant. He gave me a choice. I could either live with it as it would be unlikely to cause problems, or I could have the lump removed in a routine operation. It was my choice and I decided to have the operation. He said the scarring would be minimal and I felt peace of mind was more important. It is interesting that I was left to make the decision for myself, with no pressure from anyone. Was this a reflection of the consultant's certainty that there wasn't a serious problem? Indeed, this was reassuring, but unfortunately it gave me a rather false sense of security. I wonder what other women would have done in a similar situation? What a blessing it was that I took the decision I did.

June, and the lump was removed. I went into the day ward of my local hospital. It was here that a new discovery was made. Tests revealed that I had a congenital heart condition which could go haywire under anaesthetic. This completely shattered the illusion I had of myself being a symbol of perfect health. What an irony! The anaesthetist considered me a liability and refused to carry out a general anaesthetic. I was given a choice. I could either come back in a few days or have a local anaesthetic there and then. I opted for the latter and, although it may sound frightening, all went well and I was even able to enjoy the hospital food, unlike most of the other people in there that day!

I was told that if I heard nothing within six weeks then all was well, and I was given a date to see the consultant again in August.

After hearing nothing for more than six weeks, I checked with my local surgery who also had heard nothing; therefore, I assumed that this chapter in my life was now closed. We had a holiday booked for August and life seemed to be going well for us even though Kim was working away from home. I was busy at work and had a lively social life but now we had both decided that the time was right to plan a family. If we left it much longer, age would be against us.

August. I attended the appointment alone, feeling safe in the knowledge that this was just a routine check-up. Consequently, I was totally unprepared for the news the consultant gave me. Although the original diagnosis of a fibro-adenoma had been correct, part of the tissue that had been removed had contained cancerous cells. It appeared that there was a tumour hiding behind the fibro-adenoma! And it was purely by chance that they had happened to remove tissue that had the evidence attached to it. Suddenly I was in turmoil. On one hand I felt vindicated for making the decision to have the surgery in the first place, especially as I had not had any specific advice to do so. On the other hand, I immediately thought I was going to die. How long had I got left? The turmoil continued. My body just went weak and I became very tearful for a few minutes. After that, my mind went into overdrive. The breast care nurse was sent for and she was brilliant. I have such admiration for people like her who perform this harrowing type of nursing. She was calm, sympathetic, philosophical, reassuring and, above all, caring.

I asked question after question. I was taken for an ultrasound scan where I spent a considerable amount of time with another specialist. Despite being shocked by the news, I did manage to ask why I had not been informed of the results earlier. I never did receive a proper answer regarding this, but I was told that it was a slow-growing cancer, having a growth rate of approximately 0.2 mm per year, and that the tumour was a grade one, about 1.4 cm in size. This increased my chances of having an operation to have it completely removed.

I felt very alone at this stage, despite the hospital's efforts to help me. I finally drove home and phoned Kim, who despite his heavy workload was able to return home. By the time he arrived home, I was feeling numb and he was very subdued, little wonder. He wanted to know everything I had been told and he wanted to attempt to rationalise the situation, something he is very good at. I started to feel calmer now and began to feel more positive.

Soon I was having further tests and x-rays to check for any signs of possible secondaries, followed by more discussion. We began to feel more optimistic. It seemed that the results of all the tests were looking good. The only other area to be examined was where the lymph glands lay closest to the tumour, and this would be done during another operation to remove the tumour itself.

We were told to go off and enjoy our forthcoming holiday, if that was possible! As the cancer was slow-growing, waiting until after the holiday would make no difference.

September. And we did enjoy our holiday, despite having the knowledge of what lay ahead. I returned to hospital the Monday after we arrived back. This time I fully expected to be rid of the whole problem. After all the emotion of the initial shock I really had convinced myself that this time the operation would be successful. How wrong I was!

The operation certainly caused some consternation in the operating theatre, not to mention my 'next of kin'. Apparently, after being given the anaesthetic, my heart rate plummeted, and although I was under the care of an 'expert', I ended up in intensive care. As you could imagine, this caused real drama at home.

Eventually, when I came round, I felt perfectly fine and was totally oblivious to the monitors behind me, which, according to Kim, were performing acrobatics! He had nearly had heart failure himself upon discovering all that had happened and before he actually saw me still alive!

Thank goodness, all turned out well. My heart stabilised and I was returned to the general surgery ward where I waited for what seemed like an eternity for the results of the operation. I finally received them about four days later. But all was not well. The surgeon was not happy that he had gained sufficient clearance on all sides, and although the lymph nodes were clear, a mastectomy was suggested. This hit me like a thunderbolt. This was a far cry from a benign lump of fibrous tissue which would have left me with a 2 cm scar.

However, there appeared a little ray of hope from out of the depths. An oncologist at another hospital was consulted and he calculated that a partial mastectomy followed by radiotherapy would be sufficient treatment. Looking back, I guess I was very fortunate, although it did not feel like it at the time.

When I went home I received phone call after phone call and finally broke down when my sister called. She and Kim were a great source of strength to me. They both told me I could and would beat this thing – I just had to believe in myself.

I think my main worry was my heart. I kept thinking that I wasn't going to wake up after the next operation. I felt like I was in a catch-22 situation, damned if I had it, damned if I didn't!

This time the operation was successful. My heart held out and they gained sufficient clearance. There was some swelling afterwards and some time after a cavity appeared, which had to be regularly packed until the wound had healed. Soon I was able to start the radiotherapy. I did have reservations about this form of treatment but it was problem-free and about six months later I regained my old strength and went back to work.

The only thing was that the scar healed rather awkwardly and my breast is smaller on the left side, although people say that it is not noticeable. I have contemplated having cosmetic surgery, but there seem to be problems with this also and so for the moment I am leaving things as they are.

Right now, the only other small problem I have is my little boy, Christopher! Our long-awaited family finally arrived on 18th February, 1997, a healthy 8 lb 3 oz boy born by Caesarean section. He is a constant source of joy to us, especially as we waited so long. The traumas of the last few years are now just distant memories. We could never have imagined then that, four years on, our lives would have changed so amazingly!

And that brings us to the present. I think I am more philosophical about life now. I try not to let unimportant things become major issues. I still wonder at my chance discovery of the tumour and I'm grateful that in effect it saved my life. I know that

I have been extremely lucky and I often wonder when I hear of others who are less fortunate, *Why me?* Maybe one day I will have the answer.

Jeanette's Friend's Story

When I see my friend with her little boy, I find it hard to believe that she has had and survived breast cancer. Looking back now, at the time when it happened, I remember being shocked at the news that someone as energetic and health conscious as Jeanette should have been singled out. I've come to realise that this illness does not discriminate. My own mother, just as she hit fifty, discovered that she too had breast cancer. She has recently celebrated her sixtieth birthday and continues to enjoy good health although unfortunately has lost her husband to cancer.

I suppose we should be grateful that medical science is sufficiently advanced to help save a lot of women from radical surgery, and that there are new breakthroughs happening all the time. I am glad that Jeanette did not have to undergo a mastectomy as I know the anguish this can cause.

I would like to pay tribute to Jeanette's courage, and to all those women who work tirelessly for a better deal for breast cancer patients. The worrying fact is that, as the years go by, we all seem to know someone who has had this illness.

Chapter V
Viviane Morris

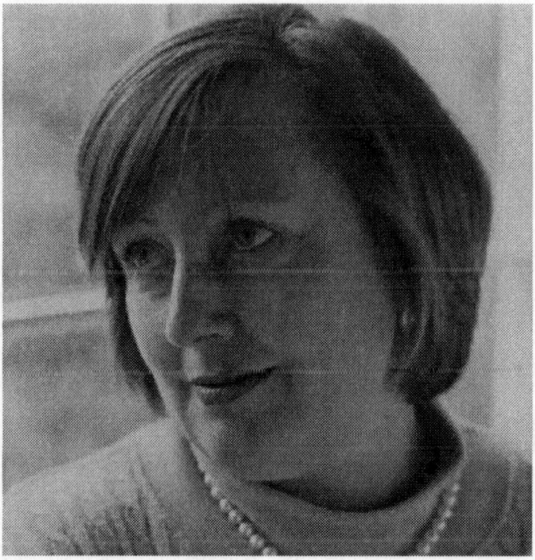

Photo by Clare Shvili, 1998

Viviane Morris lives in North London with her husband and two daughters. She had her first breast cancer in 1992 at the age of thirty-six, for which she had a partial mastectomy followed by radiotherapy. In 1997 she had a second breast cancer. Another partial mastectomy and radiotherapy followed.

Viviane's Story

Viviane was brought up in Brentwood, Essex. Her father was a well-established journalist who worked for Hansard and Lloyds List and freelanced for many of the nationals. Her mother did not work. Viviane describes her as the typical 'housewife'. She was the one who was always there for the family, while her father travelled a lot and was regularly away from home.

I was curious about the sort of diet she'd had as a youngster. She admitted that it hadn't been good: high fat with a lot of fried food. Her mother may have been unaware of nutritional values, as was typical of a lot of women of that era, but Viviane remembers that her mother always enforced the idea that you ate everything on your plate – after all, there were starving children in Africa! As a result of this, both she and her sister Valerie became overweight from an early age. She also has a younger sister, Vanessa.

Without being too personal, I asked if she'd ever taken the pill. Her reply was 'Yes', from the age of sixteen and right through to her early thirties. Really, I was trying to find out what may have caused her cancer but I soon discovered that she had a very strong view on this issue. She wrote:

> I believe that my cancer was caused by stress. I met my husband when I was thirty-one. He came from north-west London and was Jewish. We moved in together after a year or so and I converted to Judaism. His parents were very much against the situation and we had numerous problems which resulted in us getting married in St Lucia and leaving the whole family behind! It was a dreadful time for us both. I conceived Leigh, our first daughter, on our wedding

night, so when we got home and had our Jewish wedding in the synagogue I was already pregnant. Craig's parents were still not happy and we ended up not speaking for the whole of my pregnancy. However, we invited them to meet their first grandchild and our relationship has progressed very positively from there into a solid, warm and loving one.

I had given up work after the birth of Leigh, in 1990. We had bought a new home at the height of the property boom which then of course plummeted. Then, Craig was made redundant when his company folded and we lost the benefit of having a subsidised mortgage. Fortunately he found a good job quickly, but, even so, we began to struggle.

We made the decision to have a second child quickly so I could plan to return to work. I had always earned a high salary and we really needed two incomes. The mortgage rate continued to go up and our repayments became unmanageable. We began to slide into debt and although the bank was very good, the pressure was on. I have a very relaxed attitude to money when I have enough, but when I haven't I am terrified of being destitute. I seemed to spend each hour of every day panicking about how we could make ends meet and thinking through alternatives. At that time, I remember how much I wished my parents had still been alive because they would have helped us through. Instead I had no one to help and I did not want to worry Craig any more than he was already. So I bottled it all up inside and worried alone.

Once Alex was born, I knew I had to go out to work. I had let my weight increase and knew that I had to do something about that. I went to a diet doctor who gave me diet pills which I took for six months. I lost stones and I looked better than I had in years. My confidence returned and I felt that everything would be okay. And that's when I found my lump!

It was November 1992 and I was thirty-six years old. While I was having a shower one day, I checked myself and there it was.

My mother had died of bowel cancer at the age of fifty-two and my maternal grandmother had died of cancer, possibly breast cancer, at just sixty-one. I had always been aware that cancer was a threat to me but you never really imagine it happening.

I immediately telephoned the doctor. I saw an emergency GP who was particularly unpleasant. He asked me questions about the lump and said he thought it would be fine and that in view of my age, I should not worry. But he said that if I wanted to see someone then he would put me in touch. He gave me the number of a consultant whose name was familiar to me and needless to say, I phoned the next day.

I got the first available appointment in late November. The consultant was very sympathetic and tried to aspirate the lump. This was not successful and was the first real warning that all was not right. In my heart I knew it was malignant and the consultant said I'd have to have a lumpectomy.

The date for the surgery was 5th December, my third wedding anniversary. In that coming week I read literature about breast cancer and read that one in twelve women will develop breast cancer. On the day of the surgery, I couldn't help wondering who out of all the women under my consultant would be unlucky with their results.

Unfortunately it was I who was unlucky. After I had come round from the anaesthetic, the consultant confirmed my grimmest feelings that 'it did not look good', but said that we must wait for the pathology report. A few hours later it was confirmed that my tumour was indeed malignant. I felt scared, and so did everyone around me.

I was given a date for the following week to have a partial mastectomy and of course other tests to determine the stage of the cancer. My sister went with me for all the tests and gave me the moral support that I needed. My operation was scheduled for 8 a.m. on the 12th December. It was my youngest daughter's first birthday and I told the consultant that I was going to have my daughter's birthday party in my hospital room at 3 p.m.! He and the nursing staff all thought I was quite mad, but at that time I just felt I had to have this celebration in case it was the last one. Somehow, they managed to give me sufficient painkillers to enable me to get out of bed and be a part of the celebration. To watch the video film of it now is amazing as you would find it hard to believe that only five hours earlier I had been in the resuscitation room, recovering from an operation. The next day, however, I suffered, but it was worth it.

Although my husband was supportive throughout, I felt that nobody could really understand how I was feeling. I was never afraid of losing my femininity and not even worried about the scar. I have always been on the plump side and gave up bikinis in my twenties. What did concern me was my body's betrayal. Whilst I was not one for healthy food, I had never taken drugs, rarely drank and had given up smoking years before.

I hated being in hospital and kept myself occupied painting children's furniture. I worked hard at regaining the use of my arm which I had not been forewarned would be painful after the removal of the lymph nodes. The pain took a long time to pass and I have been left with a large amount of the inside of my arm completely numb. The results were encouraging, showing that the lymph glands were all clear. I then had radiotherapy treatment every day for a month. It was hard work taking two toddlers with me each day, but we managed.

I am a very positive person and am convinced that positive thoughts make a big impact on recovery after any illness. I decided that I was not going to dwell on my cancer but that instead I would get on with life. Soon after the radiotherapy, I was offered a job working for one of Craig's relatives. It sounded like fun, was local and offered me a great amount of flexibility with the children. However, in a short time the job turned into an almost full-time post and became tremendously involved. I threw myself into it, and I began earning good money which enabled us to employ a nanny to live in while I worked hard.

The job became more and more demanding, and things reached a climax during the spring of 1997. There were rumours about the company going into liquidation and that would mean redundancies. The stress became unbearable and the tensions in the office were completely out of control. Craig and I decided that we should plan for the worst. I sold my car, we moved house in order to reduce the mortgage and I let the au pair go.

The house move took place on the 12th December. Poor Alex, it was yet another spoiled birthday for her. But we made up for this by having a party a couple of days later, after which some friends came back to our new house for a celebratory drink. During the evening, I felt a pain in my breast.* Instinctively, I put my fingers over the area of pain and to my horror I could feel another lump. I think my heart stopped for a few seconds. I dived into the loo and felt under my bra. It was not my imagination – there was definitely a lump and it was big and painful. I waited until our friends had gone before telling Craig.

The consultant saw me on the Tuesday. The fact that it was a painful lump seemed to be encouraging but, once again, he could not draw any fluid off with a needle. I could tell by his face that he thought it was bad news. He hugged me, saying he was sorry but that he'd have to do another lumpectomy. Craig, who was working away in Prague, flew home for the operation which was on the very next day.

Once again, I was greeted with the bad news in the recovery room. It all seemed so unfair, I really felt that this should not be happening to me again. I had my second partial mastectomy on 30th December, 1997. The lymph nodes were clear, thankfully, but I was advised to take Tamoxifen and undergo chemotherapy. However, I spoke at great length with my oncologist and we weighed up the pros and the cons of the suggested treatment. Eventually it was agreed that neither were applicable due to the test results, so I only had radiotherapy, as before.

Within seven weeks of this last operation, I was stripping wallpaper and digging the garden! My consultant laughs at my antics and has often said he wishes he could show me off to all his other patients!

---

*(Refers to the previously unaffected breast.)

I have not returned to work. I've decided to have some time for me and my children.

At this time of writing, it is almost four months since the surgery and I am feeling happy and relaxed. I collect the children from school everyday and we are enjoying quality time together.

My real fears throughout both cancers were for my children and my husband. I cannot bear the thought of not being around for the girls during the times that they will need me. Equally, I cannot bear to think that I would not see them grow up and develop. I want to be there for them and I will be!

My husband is quiet and a man of few words, and although he was supportive, we have never discussed my cancers in great detail. We have both dealt with the situation in very different ways, but these are the only ones we know.

I beg both my sisters to check themselves regularly, but I fear they do not. They, along with my closest friends, Melanie, Sue and Marie, have been a constant source of support throughout. With each of them, I have been able to talk openly, voice my fears, and of course, cry. Each one has been touched by my cancer, and I believe it has enabled them to assess their own lives and the pressures placed upon them.

I am hoping that all the valuable lessons to be learned from my cancers will have been because I'm planning to be around for a long time to come!

Sue's Story

Viv has been a friend of mine for about ten years. We met through work and then went on to set up our own business, and even after that was sold have remained close friends through all that our lives have brought with them.

The first time she found a breast lump, I didn't believe for one moment that it would be cancer. The second time, I just knew what the result would be. Even so, when the diagnosis was confirmed, it was like a body blow, or, more accurately, a blow to the heart. I wanted to be brave and positive, if only for her, but I couldn't. It seemed like a death sentence, and when it's a close friend, there seems little else to do but cry. But I never knew whether my tears were for me, or for her, or for her two sweet, vulnerable daughters. Probably they were for all of us.

The first twenty-four hours were the worst. I couldn't stop crying and couldn't see beyond the diagnosis. All I could think was that she was too young, her children were too young. It just wasn't fair.

Ironically, it was Viv's courage that booted me out of my pessimism. Whatever she feared privately, she never showed any of us. She convinced me that this second tumour was no different to the first, that the prognosis was no worse and that she would beat it this time just like before. Eventually, I believed her.

This time I don't see it in such black and white terms. It's no longer a case of living or dying. It's more like not knowing what the future holds, but being able to live with that uncertainty.

I now feel very protective towards Viv, and I really appreciate having her around. Also, I have a great deal of respect for the way she has dealt with everything. I could only hope that in a similar situation, I would be able to find the same courage and dignity.

In the meantime, we have happily gone back to the really important issues in life: deciding which shade of green to paint the bathroom, comparing diets and of course figuring out how to dispose of four million pounds when our lottery numbers finally come up!

Chapter VI
Judith James

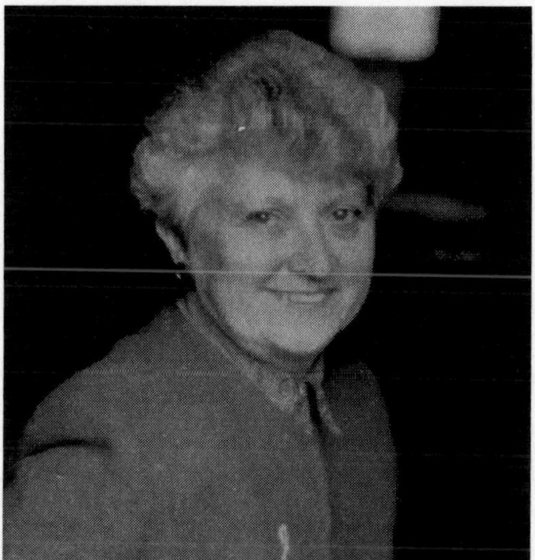

Photo by Clare Shvili, 1998

Judith James lives in Hawarden, Flintshire with her husband and has two grown-up sons. She was diagnosed with breast cancer in 1993 at the age of forty-nine. She had a mastectomy and now takes Tamoxifen.

Judith's Story

I first rang Judith when I was looking for someone to represent Wales for my book. She is one of the group contacts for Breakthrough's fund raisers. I asked Judith if she knew anyone who'd survived breast cancer and might be willing to talk to me. She said, 'Yes, me!' which took me by surprise. As it turned out, she was actually from the north of England and finally supplied me with not only her story, but also put me in touch with someone from Wales. And so, here is her story, as she told me in her letter:

> I was born in Middlesborough on 12th March, 1944, the only child of Robert and Florence Atkinson. Dad was away in India with the RAF when I was born and didn't see me until I was eight months old. We lived in the Linthorpe area of Middlesborough. Eventually my dad was invalided out of the RAF and took a job as a clerk with Cleveland Flour Mills. Mam never worked full-time after having me, but years later worked part-time collecting payments for a coal company.
>
> I went to Linthorpe Infant and Junior School, and after passing the eleven-plus examination went to Stainsby School for Girls in Acklam. After leaving school at sixteen, I began working at a local engineering company, Head Wrightson, as a commercial trainee. After five years there, I went to work in the cashiers department of our local newspaper, the *Evening Gazette*, where I stayed up until the birth of my first son, Carl.
>
> I met my husband David in May 1963 at Andy Fox and Beryl Wilson's ballroom dance studio. We were married on 24th June, 1967 in Linthorpe and bought our first house in Acklam. Carl was born on

11th February, 1970 and our second son, Simon, was born on 7th October, 1975. After eleven years we moved to Yarm, just seven miles outside Middlesborough, although my poor mum thought I was moving to the other end of the country!

Both our sons were educated in Yarm and Carl later gained a BA from Sheffield Polytechnic and an MA from Teeside Polytechnic. Simon is at present in his final year at Oxford University studying mathematics.

After living in Yarm for eighteen years, David's company, ICI, decided to move us to Hawarden in North Wales, where we live now. It was a big upheaval moving because of our families but we eventually settled down to life here.

I first noticed a lump in my left breast in July 1993. It was a Sunday evening when, getting undressed, I remarked to David that I felt bulky under my left arm. Sure enough, in the bath the next morning, I found the dreaded lump. Three days later I saw my GP who told me not to worry as he was sure it was benign because the lump was quite mobile. However, he thought that to be on the safe side, he would send me to see a consultant.

As David was in BUPA, I was able to go privately. A week later I saw the consultant. He examined me and said I had mastitis but would send me for a mammogram because of my age. A couple of days later, David and I went back for the results. We thought this was just routine, but we were shocked when the consultant said he was sorry, but there was something showing up on the mammogram that he could not ignore. It was not the original lump – this was so small and deep in my left breast that even he couldn't feel it.

Arrangements were made for me to have a lumpectomy. I had to have this done at Middlesborough General as the Nuffield had no laboratory facilities. I was on the day ward, and after the operation went back there, where I was the only patient. Fortunately David was allowed to stay with me throughout. At about 6 p.m. I was allowed to go home, even though I still had a drain in. I had to return to the hospital the next morning to have the drain removed. A few days later we went back for the results. The consultant said he was sorry to say that the tumour was cancerous, but that it was in its early stages.

To my horror, he asked me to go back to hospital the next morning for a liver scan and so, the next day, absolutely terrified, I arrived for my scan. To my relief, everything was clear, although they did find that I had gallstones! I couldn't wait to get home and phone everyone with the good news. I then had to wait for two weeks for a bone scan. My GP suggested that we go away for a few days, so David booked three nights in Paris.

After the bone scan, we returned to hospital for the results. The consultant was concerned as there were some hot spots showing up on the chest area. These actually turned out to be scarring from an accident I had had a short while before. He then went on to tell us that he was pleased with all the results, but recommended that I have a mastectomy.

Four days later, I was admitted to the Cleveland Nuffield. I had my operation at 6 p.m. and when I came round afterwards, I couldn't believe I had no pain. David visited me on his way to work the next morning and then I had a steady flow of visitors, cards and flowers. As soon as the drains were removed, I was allowed home. I was given what is called a softy prosthesis to fit in my bra until my scar healed and I could be fitted with a proper one.

The only problem that I had after the mastectomy was that my left arm was so immobile. But after the consultant explained how much tissue had been removed, I realised what the stiffness was. I was given exercises to free the stiffness, which at first were hard to do but gradually got easier. I did them religiously every day and, after about six weeks, I had the full use of my arm back.

My family and friends have been wonderful throughout and very supportive. I remember getting a bouquet from one of David's colleagues and his wife, whom I vaguely knew, and thinking, *God, I must be ill if they've sent me flowers!*

As all the nodes from under my arm were clear, no radiotherapy or chemotherapy treatment was needed and I was put on Tamoxifen. At first I was put on 40 mg per day, but in April 1995 and again in December 1995, polyps were removed from my womb, which in my case was a side effect of Tamoxifen, and the dose was reduced to 10 mg. Then in December 1997, another polyp was removed and I have now been diagnosed with fibroids, which I have been told will probably shrink down when I come off Tamoxifen, which I hope will be later in 1998.

When we moved to Hawarden, my consultant was preparing to transfer me into the care of a consultant at the Nuffield in Chester, but I had so much confidence in him that I decided to continue seeing him, and make the journey for as long as possible.

Of course, when the cancer was first diagnosed, I was upset and shed a tear. My husband feared that he might lose me and worried that the boys would have to get through their lives without a mother. My sons coped with it very well. From the very beginning I explained everything that was happening to them. They each in their own way handled the situation differently, but drew strength from my positive attitude.

I have no idea what caused the cancer. My mother didn't have breast cancer although it has come to light in the last couple of years that her eldest sister had the disease. I was on HRT for a few years, which I found great, but this hasn't been associated with my cancer.

Naturally my hopes for the future are that I continue to enjoy good health and am able to spend many more happy years with my wonderful husband David, and live long enough to see Carl and Simon settled and happy, and, of course, to become a grandma!

Judith's Father's Story

To hear of anyone having cancer is a most terrible thing, realising that some day you might lose someone you love. The trauma of that is devastating and an experience you hope will never happen. To think that my daughter had been stricken with breast cancer was quite shocking. I couldn't believe it was true; surely it couldn't happen in our family. No one had ever had this disease before.

When she told us, I was devastated and it drained me. I could not settle or put my mind to anything. My world collapsed around me and I was no good to anyone. I thought of my two grandsons: what were they going to do, how would they cope without their mother? How would Judith's husband David cope with both his own grief and that of their sons?

The day of her operation was spent clock-watching, praying and hoping they could do something to save her life. The news after was encouraging, but not conclusive. During the days after the surgery, I was living on the edge, praying that all was going to be well, and as the days went on, things were beginning to look hopeful and I felt my prayers had been answered.

Her visits to the hospital for check-ups became less frequent as each year goes by. I thank God that I have been spared the agonies of people who have lost someone close, and that today we are still together as a family.

Chapter VII
Lynne Middleton

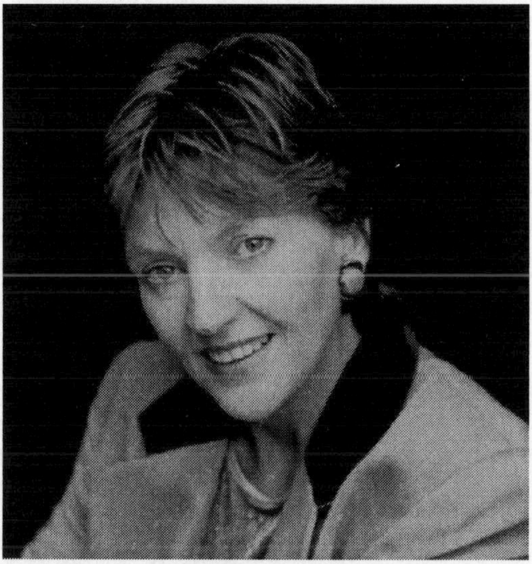

Photo by Clare Shvili, 1998

Lynne Middleton lives in Cults, Aberdeen with her husband and two children. She was diagnosed in 1997 at the age of forty-two. She had surgery, chemotherapy and radiotherapy. Now she is on Tamoxifen.

Lynne's Story

Her sense of humour is quite obvious, and she herself admits that it helped her to get through her breast cancer ordeal. She has a lovely soft Scots accent and she has very definite ideas about life. At the time of writing, it is only just over a year since she had her mastectomy but she is full of energy, always out and about doing things, as I have found out since she is never at home when I ring!

She was in her early forties when diagnosed, and this is what she wrote to me:

> I feel that I should keep my account fairly light-hearted, and, after all, my sense of humour helped get me through. If you're going to give people hope for the future, then a positive attitude towards treatment and everything else is a must.
>
> It was February 1997 when I found a lump. It was not a great shock as I had had breast problems before which had been investigated. I went through more tests and scans for my new lump, and after having a lumpectomy was told it was malignant. I had been full of hope before the operation – we were about to go on holiday to Canada for a skiing trip so my mind focused on this. I couldn't imagine anything going wrong to spoil our plans. However, we were confronted by our worst possible nightmare, and the consultant held nothing back, promising chemotherapy within days and talking immediately about a mastectomy. The holiday was definitely out the window!
>
> It was all going to happen very quickly, and I think for a while after I was perplexed and confused. My husband Neil was fantastic, however, and sort of took charge of events which helped me enormously.

We decided to tell all the family and our friends exactly what was going on, which is not pleasant. The hardest part was breaking the news to the children and my parents, but Neil did this in a very caring and positive way. The children were angry at first, presumably because our holiday had to be cancelled. My daughter, who was then aged fourteen found it particularly difficult. I could see the questions mulling around in her head… Was Mum going to die?… Will I get cancer?… How will the treatment affect Mum?… How will I cope? Thankfully she was able to answer these questions and overcome her fears by talking to her friends and even their mothers. I will be eternally grateful to all of them.

Talking to *my* friends certainly helped. I think by talking about my cancer, it actually made them feel more at ease. One thing I have never done is ask, 'Why did it happen to me?' Why not me? Years ago, for some strange reason, I used to joke with my friends about which cancer I was likely to be afflicted with, and I'd always say, 'It'll probably be my boobs! But never mind, I can always get a false pair!' Needless to say, I have stopped talking about myself in this way. In fact, I have wondered whether I actually willed it to happen,

So what did cause my cancer? Looking back, I led a fairly charmed life really. I spent a great deal of my childhood travelling abroad with my parents to far-flung places such as India and Pakistan. Schooling was in Aberdeen at an all-girls' school, and then at college where I graduated in dress and textiles. Then, after college, I took a year out to follow my parents to Adelaide and did a secretarial course to pass the time away. When I returned to Aberdeen, I had several office jobs with a variety of oil companies which I thoroughly enjoyed.

There was no pressure, no stress and I had a fabulous circle of friends. I finally settled down to married life at the age of twenty-four and continued to work until our daughter was born four years later. Around this time I decided to stop smoking and I have wondered if smoking, and drinking too much alcohol in my youth, contributed to the cancer. But then, I also have to consider the contraceptive pill, hormone-injected factory chickens, red meats, ingestion of potentially lethal chemicals in food and, of course, stress, which can all possibly play their part in causing illness, certainly in producing side effects. I once read somewhere that stress exists only in the mind and yet we know it is a killer.

But getting back to my treatment… After I'd started my chemo, the worst thing to happen was that I lost my hair. It's a real give-away about your illness – people do notice when an eyebrow drops off! I held on to my hair for as long as possible but eventually decided to ask my hairdresser to shave my head as the hair was starting to fall out in handfuls and the tiny follicles were tender.

Looking into the mirror was the hardest part, but once the wig was in place I looked fine. Admittedly, though, some evenings when I was getting ready to go out, I did feel a bit like I was dressing up in drag! False eyelashes, painted eyebrows and all manner of flamboyant hats and scarves. Things which frightened me then were high winds, umbrellas, low branches and babies with wandering hands! Would the wig stay on?

It was difficult concealing my temporary baldness from the children. I used to go to extraordinary lengths, even at the swimming pool, just to appear normal for their sakes. I even climbed a mountain in the middle of summer, donning a wig and hat!

I now believe that I've beaten the disease. I've come through the chemotherapy, mastectomy and radiotherapy, although none of this could have been achieved without a very caring husband, a brilliant surgeon, the superb back-up care I received and of course all my family and friends who really believed that I could beat the cancer.

My positivenesss came mainly from meeting other patients in hospital who urged me to listen to a chap called Jack Black who is a motivational speaker. His ideas about personal development, meditation for calmness and correct positive thinking were just what I was looking for.

You need to call upon your reserves for those terrible black moments and to manage your stress levels so that you can take control of your life. I read every single article I could find about breast cancer. I wanted to know about every new treatment, complementary medicine etc., and I think I drove the doctors mad with all my infernal questions. But I have to say that they answered every one and the oncology unit provided fantastic support for Neil and myself.

Now I want to put all this behind me and really start living each day to the full, trying to forget about unimportant things which would have bothered me before. I would also like to help others in a similar situation and be able to say, 'Hi guys! There is light at the end of the tunnel!'

I would also like to say thanks in some small way by fund-raising for the hospital. In fact we have just managed to raise two thousand five hundred pounds from a dance that we organised.

It is impossible to cover all aspects of my treatment, worries and fears, but I do remember thinking during chemo that I must keep myself incredibly fit. I also drank gallons of aloe vera gel and swallowed handfuls of vitamin pills in the hope that I could help my failing immune system to regain its proper working order.

For the moment I cannot imagine having a reconstruction done as it's still early days. So for the meantime I have to manage the false boob. I tell my friends to look out for the creeping shoulder pad as it might just be something else! (It doubles as a duster by the way!)

And finally, we did manage to have that skiing holiday after all, three months after my mastectomy. It was worth waiting for!

Lynne's Friend's Story

We have been friends since primary school. We went to the same college and have kept in close contact during the last twenty years.

I have been in awe of her ever since the day I found out about her breast cancer. This sweet, caring, loyal friend has become a warrior. Hidden to me in the past is an inner strength which has helped Lynne through. From day one, she has searched for ways to make this difficult journey a more comfortable one. She attended positive-thinking courses, sought out the best diet and walked miles and miles! In fact all of her friends are so envious of the way she looks that we are beginning to try some of the things Lynne discovered.

Breast cancer is not all doom and gloom. Lynne has shown me that you *can* make a difference to this frightening disease by not giving in to it.

Chapter VIII
Linda Jacoby

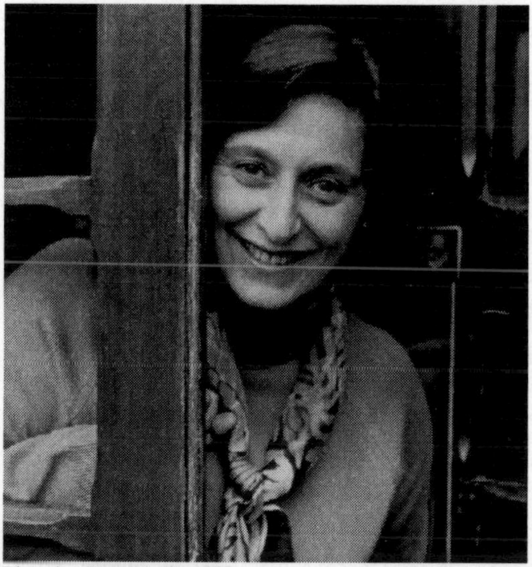

Photo by Clare Shvili, 1998

Linda Jacoby lives in Maidenhead, Berkshire with her husband and two teenage daughters. Her breast cancer was diagnosed in 1995 when she was forty-two. She had surgery followed by radiotherapy and is now taking Tamoxifen.

Linda's Story

Linda phoned me one Sunday afternoon to say she was interested in contributing to my book. I was in the middle of chaos, as usual, and she took me a little by surprise. As she gave me a brief outline of her experience, I listened intently. Her openness astonished me, but then again, why shouldn't she have been open?

She told me that she had grown up in North London – the accent was still there although quite mellow. She came from a working class family, and was brought up as a Christian. Although she was not dismissive about her past, the real focus of her life now is her family. She spoke lovingly and proudly of her two daughters, Sarah and Rachel.

'Very Jewish names,' I commented.

'Oh yes,' she replied, 'their father is Jewish, but they are brought up to have an open religious understanding of the world.' Linda was very adamant about that.

After receiving her letter a short time after this, I realised that any questions I had asked about different possible trigger factors from her past were really not applicable. Stress was the probable cause, if it could ever be proved.

Her story is honest and to the point. The following is what she wrote:

> I suppose, looking back, it all started in 1990. At thirty-seven years old, suddenly I found that I was feeling very tired. I would become exhausted after doing the hoovering and would have to sleep for an hour after lunch. To begin with, I put it down to being a full-time mum and housewife, part-time swimming teacher and 'chauffeur' to the girls. On top of which, I was married to a workaholic who was constantly on the move with his job.

But after about six months, I was concerned enough to visit my doctor who sent me for a series of tests – thyroid, heart, hormone balance. All of these proved negative, which led the young registrar I'd seen at the hospital to suggest that I was suffering from 'housewives' syndrome' and I ought to take up a few more hobbies! The cheek of it, I ask you!

The problem didn't get any better. In 1992 my husband's job took us to Strasbourg, which while very exciting and enjoyable, was also extremely stressful. Coping with another language and culture with two children and a husband travelling four days a week wasn't easy. I was lonely as well as tired all the time. I began eating all the wrong things, such as chocolate and the lovely French pastries. I found after a while that I was using food to give me a boost of energy in order to get me through the day, and despite exercising three times a week, I was gradually putting on weight and feeling worse and worse.

Eventually in 1994 we returned to the UK, and it was in the November that I noticed a very painful lump in my left breast. I was slightly worried and had it checked. It turned out to be a benign cyst that was already going down, but I was sent for a mammogram as a precautionary measure. The x-ray showed up two unusual spots, so I then had an ultrasound scan and luckily everything was okay.

I had regular check-ups over the next six months, and then I found another lump high up in the left breast. Several needle aspirations were carried out, all of which proved to be negative. In July 1995, I saw the consultant. He said I could choose whether or not to have this second lump removed and gave me until September to decide.

Over the summer, I found myself often rubbing this area as it was uncomfortable. By the September, I had decided to have the lump removed. This was done under local anaesthetic, although it proved to be much deeper than had originally been anticipated. Funnily enough, I remember commenting to my husband a couple of days later how much better I felt in myself.

A week later I returned to see the surgeon. He greeted me with the words, 'I think you had better sit down. I have some bad news for you.' I had a malignant tumour! Although it was a shock, I found that I was relatively calm. I felt a sense of relief somehow. After all this time, the tiredness and the tests, at last the reason why had been discovered. Even the consultant seemed surprised at my reaction, but for him it was probably a lot easier to deal with than to be faced with someone deeply traumatised or made hysterical by the news.

I went to find a phone and telephoned my husband. Then I made my way home – I cried all the way. As soon as I got in, I confronted my daughters with what had happened. They were shocked, but I emphasised that I'd *had* cancer, and whatever treatment was to follow, was purely preventative.

Ten days later, I was back in hospital for a second operation. This was to remove a wider section of breast tissue close to where the lump had been, to ensure that there were no stray cancer cells. The lymph nodes from under my arm were also removed to check for possible spread of the disease. I was in hospital for ten days rather than the usual three or four. The reason for this was that we were having some building work done at home and everyone was worried that with the breast drains still in place, I would be prone to infection from the amount of dust in the air.

Five days after the operation, the results of the tissue samples came back. The lymph nodes were all clear! So, once the drains were removed and already taking Tamoxifen, I went home. Three days later I saw the oncologist who explained what further treatment I would have. She also explained that there was a trial underway trying to establish the best combined treatment for breast cancer. If I agreed to take part in the trial, I might either have chemotherapy and radiotherapy, or radiotherapy and Tamoxifen, or any one of these on their own, or nothing at all!

This led to a family conference around the kitchen table. Everyone had their say and then a family decision was made. Although I was keen to help medical knowledge, we decided that if I didn't need chemotherapy then I wouldn't take part in the trial and would just have radiotherapy and continue with Tamoxifen.

About a month later, I attended the radiotherapy unit in the hospital, where I was tattooed with a marker pen to outline the areas for the treatment. The following week I started the six week course of radiotherapy.

This became very much a routine – same time, same place – and for the first two or three weeks I didn't feel any side effects. But then I noticed that as each day went by, I was gradually starting to feel more tired. During the last week, the 'sunburnt' effect that had developed over the weeks became uncomfortable and this in turn made movement difficult.

For a period afterwards, I saw the consultant and the oncologist alternately every three months. Now, my check-ups are annual, but I'm still taking Tamoxifen.

I suppose the obvious question that people will ask is how did I feel while all this was going on, and how do I feel now?

Once the initial relief of knowing what was wrong with me had worn off, the only thought in my head was for my children. I decided that there was no way that I would finish being their mum, and possibly miss out seeing them grow up and perhaps go to University or get married. My eyes and my heart were firmly fixed on the horizon.

I described it to my breast care counsellor as like being on a train journey, where I had to make damn sure that I got off at my station. I also phoned BACUP, who were really helpful and reassuring. They explained things very clearly to me, which helped me a lot, and they also praised the way that I had told my children. They also sent me lots of literature, which, as a family, helped us to come to terms with what had happened.

People have described me as strong, courageous, and most of all incredibly positive. But to be honest, I don't think I was any of those things. It was purely and simply my way of dealing with the situation. I felt as though I'd been very lucky and would do whatever was needed to survive. This was not going to be the end of my life; I wasn't ready to curl up and die, not yet! I was also very aware of the effect my attitude would have on my two girls. I wanted them to understand that cancer was a disease that you could recover from and not necessarily something to be afraid of.

And although they were obviously shocked and frightened to begin with, on the whole, they took it well. I tried hard to involve them in my treatment, taking them to radiotherapy to see how it all worked. Most of all though, I've just tried to be honest with them.

My husband was different, though. He has always had a strong fear of cancer and so found it very hard to cope with in the beginning. When I was first diagnosed, he was devastated, and even now he finds it difficult to allow himself to believe that I have survived and that the cancer won't come back. My parents were also badly affected. Their generation viewed cancer almost as a 'mysticism' and, even now, they are very frightened for me.

I feel very lucky to have had such caring and supportive friends. Lots of people phoned, visited and sent flowers – I was overwhelmed and very touched. It all helped me to stay positive. One friend who was training to become a homeopath sent me lots of remedies to help with different stages of my treatment. As she had recently lost a close relative to cancer, she had lots of books about positive thought and so on, and she kept nagging me to take things easy and rest properly. Other friends couldn't believe it had happened. One friend used to send me funny cards at odd intervals just to cheer me up and let me know that she was thinking of me. Several others kept close tabs on me to make sure I did what I was supposed to do! I think that knowing people care about you is a very important part of recovery.

Of course, it's not all easy. Whenever there's an unexplained ache or pain, I do wonder. But as far as I'm concerned, the future will be long and fulfilling. The cancer has had a positive effect on my life. It has made me re-evaluate. I realised the importance of a healthy diet and its role in preventing cancer. I have changed my diet and I've now lost three stones in weight which makes me feel great.

Life is too short and I've decided to try and do all the things that I've always wanted to. It's also made me put my house in order – I try not to leave anything until tomorrow. But the most important lesson that I've learned, is that cancer can be beaten.

Life is a very precious thing and it needs to be lived to the full, *now*!

Linda's Daughter's Story

I was fifteen when the doctors found that my mum had breast cancer. I had never expected anything like this to happen. Your parents always appear to be invincible, people whom no one can harm.

I knew Mum was stressed because my dad was away on business so much. While we were living in France, the stress increased as Dad was still away a lot and my sister and I were finding it difficult to settle into our new lifestyle.

The thing that surprised me the most was that Mum was never ill. Even when the rest of the world was flu ridden, she was okay.

She and my dad kept all the tests a secret from us, until they knew the lump was malignant, and in some ways it was good because I would have been really worried. However, the fact that I had never suspected anything made the truth even more horrifying. I remember being told and I immediately began to well up with the shock and horror.

I was not horrified at my mum having cancer, but more by the fact that something so awful could happen to someone so kind, and to someone who was never ill. At first, I felt anger towards my father because of the problems his work had created. But once Mum's treatment had started, my anger subsided and I began to have different feelings. During the treatment, I was afraid to touch her in case I hurt her. Visiting in hospital was also very difficult as she looked so vulnerable, not the way I was used to seeing her.

Then I saw her gain an inner strength, which, to this day, I truly admire. Nothing was going to stop her conquering this and she continually asked for our support which we were all happy to give.

I think this has changed my attitude to life. I will always use her as my example because I don't know anyone more courageous. I hope that I will be able to teach my children to have this sort of courage in life, and I hope *she* will be able to teach them to live each day to the full.

Chapter IX
Jo Evans

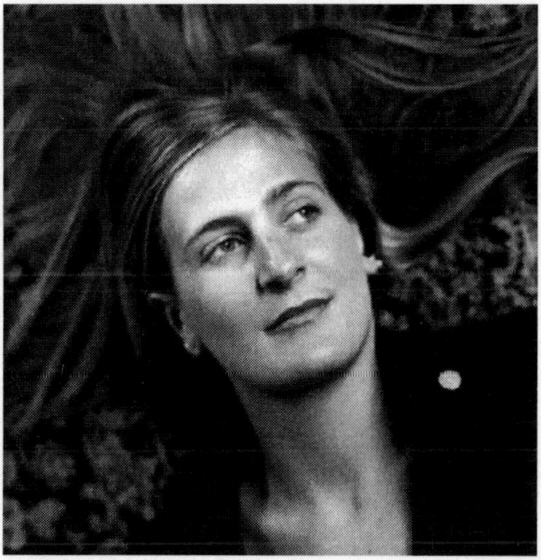

Photo by Clare Shvili, 1998

Jo Evans lives with her boyfriend in Liverpool. She was diagnosed with breast cancer in 1997 when she was in her mid-twenties. She had surgery followed by radiotherapy and has been on Tamoxifen ever since.

Jo's Story

When I spoke to Jo on the telephone, I had quite a shock! I was expecting a broad Liverpudlian accent but only if you really bend your ear can you detect a slight twang of the neighbourhood!

After listening to Jo's story, it makes you wonder how such a thing can happen to a lovely young girl, but it must be emphasised at this point that to have breast cancer in your mid-twenties is very uncommon. But, by the same token, it's not unheard of.

Of course, you can't fail to be moved by her story, as indeed I was. After receiving her draft and reading it, I cried buckets, partly because it reminded me of my own situation and emotions, and partly because I felt like I wanted to give her a big hug! But it has to be said that there is light at the end of the tunnel.

It is such an honest account that I prefer to use her own words:

> I was born 6th December, 1971 in Liverpool. I have a brother and sister both younger than myself. We have always lived in Liverpool apart from a year when my father got a job in Sweden, but I was too young to remember that.
>
> I went to Huyton College for girls, from the age of four right up until my A levels. I suppose I was an average student – hard working, enjoying sport and making some good friends. To me, school was fun, and I was captain of the first lacrosse team. I also enjoyed tennis, swimming, diving and rounders.
>
> As a family, we were quite fortunate. Every January we went skiing and in the summer we either went to France or visited family in America. My mother and father are both doctors, my brother is a

law student and my sister is studying aeronautical engineering. We are an extremely close 'fivesome', along with our two Scottie dogs!

After deciding that I wasn't bright enough for university, I decided to carve out a career in banking. Eventually, after applying to all the banks, the Royal Bank of Scotland offered me a job which I started soon after my final exams.

I met my boyfriend Andy at work more than four years ago. I can tell him anything and we've shared a lot of laughter and tears during our time together. I have many friends, but four in particular, Julie, Liz, Lucy and Joanne, along with Andy and of course my family, were the real driving force behind my recovery from the Big 'C'.

It's not that I can't say or use the word cancer, but the Big 'C' is what my parents have always called it. In the past, I understood it as always being associated with death and meaning bad news. Young people didn't get cancer; people whose lives hadn't quite taken off didn't get cancer; healthy people who didn't smoke, ate carefully and played lots of sport didn't get cancer… or did they? This was my ignorant opinion, but now I know differently. Cancer does not discriminate.

So it was March 1997 and I noticed a small hard bump in my chest, just left of my breast. I thought it must be a cyst or a hardening of tissue. I kept touching it for three weeks before I mentioned it to Andy. He told me to get my mum to have a look but I decided to put it off – it would surely go away.

In May of that year, Andy and I went off to Spain to visit his parents who were out there. The whole week we were there, I became obsessed with feeling the 'bump'. It wasn't growing and only hurt when I pressed it, but Andy insisted that I should get it sorted out when we got home. I will never forget – it was Sunday, 11th May when I talked to Mum about it. She was confident that everything would be okay, but even so thought I should see the GP. As I got ready for bed that evening, my stomach was in knots. My dad had noticed that I was not myself and he tried to reassure me.

On the Monday afternoon I went to the GP who examined me and arranged an appointment for me at the Royal Liverpool University Hospital Breast Assessment Clinic on Thursday, May 15th. This became known as D-Day, diagnosis day!

When I went, it was a glorious sunny day. I remember sitting in the car while I was waiting to go in and the radio was playing Robbie Williams singing *I Hope I'm Old Before I Die.* This song haunted me for the next six months.

I must say, as I have been asked many times, the fact that my parents are doctors, had no influence on the treatment I received. I was just lucky enough to live close to an assessment centre and this was really the greatest benefit.

I sat alone in the waiting room and was given a sheet explaining the procedures. I was called quite quickly and was given a shopping basket to put my clothes in after changing into one of those 'hideously difficult to tie' robes. I was then examined and, because the lump was so small, I was to have an ultrasound scan and a fine needle aspiration. I don't care what anyone says – the needle hurt! Then I was asked to get dressed and wait.

Judging by the other patients waiting with me, I was, without doubt, the youngest at twenty-five, and I wanted my mum! I had arranged to meet my dad afterwards as he worked at this hospital. After thirty-five minutes, I heard the nurse telephoning him to make sure that he could come to a room where there was a big pink sofa with fluffy cushions and at that moment it suddenly dawned on me that the results were not good.

At exactly 3.04 p.m. I was told that my lump was cancerous. One minute later my dad entered the room. His worried eyes locked with mine as tears streamed down my face. He wept and all I remember saying to him was, 'Daddy, I've got cancer, am I going to die?' The surgeon and the breast care nurse both explained what was going to happen next. They were going on about blood tests, surgery, results and radiotherapy, but I was in no fit state to take it all in. I kept shaking and asking, 'Will I die? Will I be able to have kids? Will I lose my breast?' None of my questions were in any kind of order and soon Dad was leading me to the car. While he drove us home, I hardly took my eyes off him.

When we got home, we sat in the lounge. I was still shaking, crying and praying. I couldn't think straight but I remember feeling compelled to ring everyone I knew and tell them. We had to wait two hours before Mum arrived home as we had decided not to phone her with such bad news. When she got in, we just ran up to her and she hugged us both even though she still hadn't been told the news. My mum was very practical and optimistic about the whole thing. She wanted to know when the surgery would be and what happened next.

There was a very definite order of events for the next few weeks. The surgery would take place in two weeks, followed by the results after another two weeks, and finally I would have the required treatment. Looking back, I think this helped me to deal with each step, and understand what was happening.

Andy came over later, and I found it very hard breaking the news to him. I said to him that I would understand if he wanted us to split but he was horrified at my suggestion and I immediately regretted it. That night, my dad slept in my bedroom with me, and we talked about anything and everything until the small hours.

The following Monday, the breast care nurse came to see me at home. In my mind, I was hoping that she had come to tell me the whole thing had been a big mistake, but in reality she explained about my surgery, drew a diagram to help me understand better and gave me some leaflets to read. She told me that I would have a blood test and chest x-ray a week before my operation.

It was strange going into hospital on a lovely summer's day and when I was feeling so well. I was visited by the ward consultant, the surgeon and a lady who was doing research on the care breast cancer patients receive. I can't tell you how wonderful the nurses were. From the moment I arrived, right through to my recovery, they were fantastic.

At 6 a.m. the next morning, a nurse woke me up and I was allowed a cup of tea and some toast. I got up, had a shower and watched breakfast television. My dad came to see me at 8.15 a.m. on his way to a meeting. I still had over three hours to kill before they wheeled me off so I was glad of the distraction. Just as he was leaving, I burst into tears and told him I was scared. He gave me a hug as only a dad can do.

Shortly after, the anaesthetist came along to see me followed by the house officer. They asked me whether I had any questions, which I didn't, and proceeded to mark me up for surgery with a marker pen. I was given a delightful pair of surgical stockings to put on but the pièce de résistance had to be the string knickers I was expected to wear!

An hour later I was being wheeled down to theatre. I waited on the trolley in a room with several other patients waiting for surgery. There was an elderly man opposite me who was about to have a major operation. He was laughing and joking with the staff and as I knew that my operation wasn't nearly as bad as his, this thought gave me the strength I needed to get through. It was 12.45 p.m. as the anaesthetist put me into the land of nod.

When I came round, I was in the recovery room feeling groggy. It wasn't long before I was taken back to my room and I must have drifted off to sleep because the next time I woke it was about 5 p.m. I was suddenly aware of all the tubes that were attached to me and I couldn't move my left side. During the next few hours I felt pretty rough.

By Saturday lunchtime, the day after surgery, I felt much better, and although my left side was very stiff, there wasn't a great deal of pain. The nurses showed me how the drains worked and told me that as soon as I felt strong enough to go to the toilet by myself, I must carry the drains and not pull them. They put the bottles at the end of the drains into a plastic carrier bag which made it slightly easier for me. When my sister came to visit me later and saw me walking around clutching the bag, she said I looked like an old 'bag woman'!

I left hospital on the Monday morning, both drains having been removed. I felt rather delicate and a bit light-headed. In the next few days, my parents took me out for nice lunches and we tackled the

Times Two crossword most days to keep our minds distracted.

The night before my results, Dad and I stayed up for most of the night watching banal television. We spoke only briefly about what the doctors could or could not say, but we decided it was best not to ponder and wait.

The next day, both my parents went with me to get the results. We were told that the tumour had been grade two and about the size of a pea. But the really good news was that there was no spread to the lymph nodes! I felt sick with relief and my eyes wetted with tears. I was told that I would be having just radiotherapy treatment for five weeks and hormonal therapy in the form of Tamoxifen which I would have to take for the next five years.

I went to Clatterbridge Hospital for the radiotherapy, which took me forty minutes' travel time each way. This in itself tired me out. I would usually have a rest after I got home from the hospital, and then afternoons would be taken up with either phone calls from friends and colleagues, receiving faxes from my friend Lucy who was touring Australia and the States, and visits to every art gallery, museum and garden centre in Merseyside!

I went back to work part-time after my last radiotherapy session and started back full-time in the October. I am now well used to taking the Tamoxifen and so far the only problems that I have had have been the hot flushes, or power surges as my Dad calls them!

I wouldn't say the experience has changed the whole of my life, but I certainly do take my own health very seriously and not for granted like before. I can't blame any one thing for what has happened and

I may never find out what caused my cancer. My biggest fear is that the cancer may return, but I regularly examine myself and have three monthly check-ups.

Of course, nobody can tell me what will happen, but after counselling I have realised that I mustn't dwell on things. I admit that I have my bad days, but I've also learnt not to bottle things up and find having a good cry really helps. I still have flashbacks to the time of my diagnosis and I still get upset if I read accounts of other people's experiences or watch a TV programme about breast cancer, although afterwards, I usually feel a stronger person.

On the positive side, I feel physically fit, am very happy with Andy and plough all my spare energies into breast cancer awareness and fund-raising!

Jo's Friend's Story

May 1997. I had just returned from a week abroad when one of my closest friends telephoned, for what I thought would be a general 'welcome home' chat and update on the latest gossip.

How wrong I was. The ensuing conversation brought about some of those emotions that you hope there won't be many of in life.

At first I remained silent. Then came the tears and with them shock, fear, dread and confusion. Cancer in one so young, I thought? What next? How could I help and what did she need from her friends? How were her family coping?

Although we had only been friends for a couple of years, we were very close. We shared the same sense of humour and enjoyed a good shop!

Following the news, I wanted so much for Jo to know how much I cared for her. Of course I sent her cards and flowers, but I felt that the most I could give was just to be there for her when she needed me. I visited and tried to make her laugh, and when she needed to we talked about the future, her treatment and the daunting operation, which I know she was fearful about. But when the time came, she found the courage and inner strength to hold herself together.

Cancer is a word that I associate with the old. Jo was young and happy which made me feel helpless and frustrated. The most I could do was offer support and listen when the need arose. Thankfully I have remission myself in knowing that Jo is well and in the main, back to her old self; however, now and again the hurt returns whenever cracks in her armour appear.

Keep well Jo, and always know that 'You've got a friend'.

Chapter X
Jean Hurd

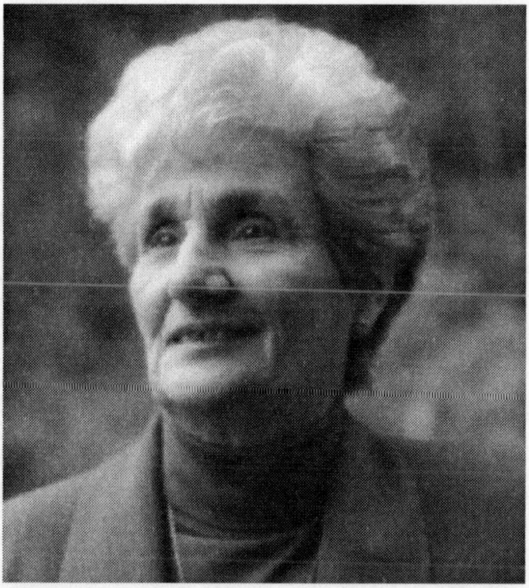

Photo by Clare Shvili, 1998

Jean Hurd lives near to Cheadle Cheshire. She is widowed, has two grown-up daughters and two grandchildren. She was diagnosed with breast cancer in 1993 when she was in her fifties. She had surgery and radiotherapy and was prescribed Tamoxifen.

Jean's Story

There is a real irony to Jean's story. I met Jean through her daughter Julie. Julie and I were both converting to Judaism, and were on the same course. I will never forget, it was Passover, which usually falls around Easter time. It was a Saturday morning and we were all at synagogue. After the service, as usual, everyone got together for a chinwag and a bit of finger food. After most people had left, Julie calmly told us that her mum had just been diagnosed with breast cancer. As she spoke the words, I felt a surge of heat gush through my body. These were words of dread for me. As we stood there talking, unbeknown to anyone, I too was harbouring a tumour in my breast, and, indeed, two months later I would also be diagnosed with the same disease.

It was a very difficult moment, trying to concentrate on what Julie was telling me and yet at the same time trying not to make comparisons. Of course, we have both come through it, and we have kept in contact over the ensuing years, during the good times and the bad. For both of us, there have been other elements to our ordeals, and for all these reasons I could not have left Jean out of this book.

To write about Jean on her own, if you know her, just doesn't sound right. It's a bit like writing about Morecombe without Wise. I am of course referring to the absence of her husband, Norris, who tragically died only a few years ago, from cancer. I know that if she could dedicate this piece to anyone, it would be to 'Norrie'.

Jean was born in Salford, an only child, just a few years before the Second World War broke out. Sadly, her mother died from peritonitis in 1939 when Jean was only four. Her childhood was very disruptive, mainly due to the war, and she ended up living with different relatives on and off during the Blitz. After the war, she returned to Salford to live with her father and grandma.

She left school at fifteen and went to work as a clerk in a textile company in Manchester. She met Norris on her sixteenth birthday – some present! Three years later they were married. Michelle, their eldest daughter, arrived on the scene four years later, and Julie after a gap of six years. They were a close and happy family, and apart from Jean having a gallstone removed in 1972, they had both remained in good health.

Then, in 1993, Jean went for her first routine mammogram. It was Tuesday, 21st February and she had to go to a mobile unit at Steppinghill Hospital. It was a sunny day and she felt fine. Three days later, a letter arrived saying that the result of the x-ray was unclear and that they now wanted her to go to the Nightingale Centre at Withington Hospital for another mammogram.

By this time she was starting to feel a little uneasy. When Norris came home that night, she told him and they sat and discussed the situation, eventually deciding to keep everything to themselves to save worrying their girls.

Norris went with Jean on the day. The staff were more than welcoming and tried to reassure them that recalls were usually because the original x-rays were difficult to read. After a while, Jean went for the mammogram and then waited approximately fifteen minutes until a doctor came. He told her that the x-ray was showing a white patch, and he wanted her to have an ultrasound scan which would give a clearer picture of what was going on.

She was taken into another room for the scan, and the white patch now clearly showed up as a small tumour. Everyone remained quite calm and Norris was asked to go into the room where Jean was. She briefly explained what was going on before the consultant came. He was a quiet-spoken person, and he showed them the x-ray plates and scan pictures, explaining as he went along. He wanted to perform a needle biopsy there and then, which he did, saying that he was fairly sure that the lump was malignant.

I must interject here – to the reader, this may seem a shocking way to worry someone into believing they have cancer, but I personally feel that a realistic approach is far better than leading the patient into a false sense of security.

Jean was understandably numb with shock at the consultant's words. Here she was, feeling so well and yet being faced with the possibility of a life-threatening disease. She was advised to have a lumpectomy and was told to expect to receive an appointment within the next few days.

A week passed and no appointment was arranged. So she rang the Nightingale Centre who said that all her notes had been sent to Wythenshawe Hospital, where she was to have the operation, and advised calling there. She managed to speak to the consultant's secretary but was told that they too had not got Jean's notes and therefore didn't know anything about what was going on!

By now, the worry had turned to anger. In her own mind, the tumour was growing daily. But it took several more phone calls and some pestering before she was told that an appointment had been arranged for the consultant's next clinic. Her relief at this was immense. The family and her close friends, now knowing the full implications, offered their support and Jean was surrounded by warm, caring people.

Soon she was off to the hospital again with Norris to see the consultant. He examined her and said she was down for his next day in theatre. The staff told her to be as positive as she could be, which in my opinion is the only way to be.

Not long after, she was in hospital having the lumpectomy. She was just in for a few days and started taking Tamoxifen straight after the surgery. A week later, she returned to hospital for the results. Yes indeed, it was cancer, and she was being transferred to the Christie Hospital, renowned for its cancer treatments. There she would have fifteen sessions of radiotherapy treatment, and that was all.

Jean's mental attitude was getting stronger, but Norris was still worried and found the whole illness difficult to cope with. I think the partner is always at a disadvantage for they can only watch what is happening to their loved one, and probably feel a sense of uselessness. In this way, Norris just wanted everything to get back to normal and Jean to feel her old self once again.

The only side effect from the treatment was tiredness, which seemed to Jean to last for ages, but, as she said, it's a small price to pay for saving your life.

When she had finally regained her strength, she went to the GP for a routine smear test. To her complete shock, the results showed irregular cells. What next? She was referred to the gynaecologist back at Wythenshawe Hospital, who suggested laser treatment, a D&C and a biopsy. She waited about two weeks for an appointment on the day ward. As usual, Norris was with her every step of the way, and once it was all over, they hoped that this would be the last of the problems.

But as fate would have it, that was not to be. Six months later, another smear revealed the same irregular cells. And then there was another blow. Jean found another lump, this time in her other breast. Again, both had to be operated on, and the two surgeons decided to operate on the same day. This done, Jean received the good news that the lump in her breast had turned out to be no more than a cyst, and with the cervix problem treated, she could get back to normal.

Although it took her a few months to feel fully recovered, life seemed to be getting back on track. Jean and

Norris's fortieth wedding anniversary was approaching, and Michelle and Julie started organising a party.

Then fate dealt yet another blow. It was only a couple of weeks until the Ruby Wedding celebrations, July 1994. Jean noticed a lump on Norris's back and persuaded him to go to the doctor. When he did, the doctor remarked on how well he looked, but, however, examined him from top to toe. Jean was there with Norris when the doctor told him that his liver was enlarged, which gave cause for concern. Jean had a feeling that things were not good. Seven days later, they learned that he had lung and liver cancer.

Listening to Jean tell this story, you know that this overshadowed all her own previous health problems. She just couldn't understand how someone could look so fit and healthy, yet conceal such dreadful disease.

At Norris's own request, the party was to go ahead without anyone other than the immediate family knowing about his illness. It was hard, but they had a lovely time. I had to laugh when Jean said, 'They get Oscars for that kind of acting in Hollywood!' One can only imagine how difficult it must have been.

Sadly, in October 1994, Norris died. Jean had lost her 'soulmate'. She is still devastated by his death, and admits that she feels guilty that she has survived when he didn't.

She is now more than six years down the line from the cancer, and although life is hard without Norris, she faces a future surrounded by her loving family.

I know myself that the pain of losing a loved one is very hard, and I think that losing your lifelong partner must be even more difficult. However, with the passage of time, coping and learning to live with your loss gets easier. I hope that is the case for Jean, because she's still got a lot of living, and loving, left to do!

Jean's Daughter Michelle's Story

After reading my mum's account of her breast cancer, I felt that reading it in a few short paragraphs seemed to minimise how much cancer affects the patient and his or her family and friends.

I remember this period of time as a photographic diary.

The first picture I remember is a grey February morning. I am holding my eighteen-month-old daughter by a window at home, waiting for Mum and Dad to come from the Nightingale Centre, the local breast cancer treatment centre. When they arrive, they tell me that the lump is malignant and explain what the treatment will be. At this point, it is hard to put into words how I felt.

The second picture is of Dad and me walking down a corridor of Wythenshawe Hospital on the day of Mum's lumpectomy. I remember trying to comfort Dad because he looked grey with worry and concern. I remember feeling that now the lump had been removed, we were one step nearer to getting Mum healthy again. The day after the operation I visited Mum. She told me that the consultant had been to see her and had prescribed Tamoxifen, which also gave me a feeling of optimism.

The next step was the radiotherapy at the Christie Hospital. I was so grateful to all our family and friends who rallied round to take Mum for her daily treatment.

Mum has just reached six years cancer-free and is officially in remission. I want to take this opportunity to say how much I admire her strength and determination, and I know how strong she has been for all of us.

Just before Mum and Dad's Ruby Wedding in 1994, Dad was diagnosed with lung and secondary liver cancer, and although he fought the disease, sadly he died in October the same year. We were all devastated, especially

Mum, as they were soulmates and very much in love.

I want to finish by saying how much *I love my mum* and how grateful I am that she is once again healthy.

Chapter XI
Julia Wolfe

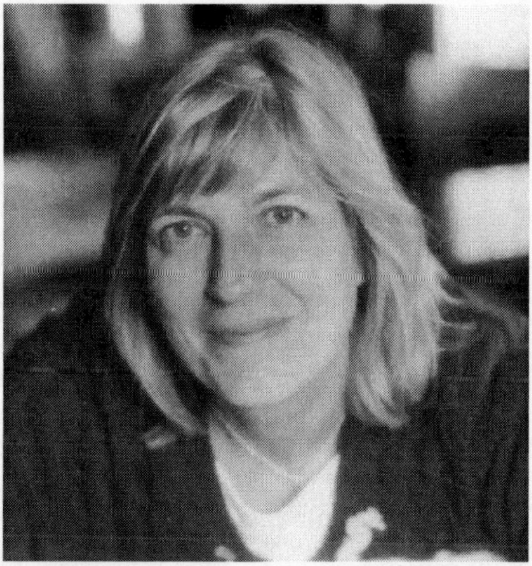

Photo by Clare Shvili, 1998

Julia Wolfe lives in London with her husband and two young children. She had breast cancer in 1995 when she was in her mid-thirties. She had surgery, chemotherapy, radiotherapy, and given Tamoxifen.

Julia's Story

When Julia sent me her story, there was a letter attached to it which said, 'I have written a screed, very quickly and without analysing it too much. No doubt you will lick it into shape!' But when I read it, written quickly or not, it was so well done that I could not possibly try to improve upon it. Her writing is interesting and articulate, a bit like her personality I would imagine, although at the time of writing I have only spoken with Julia on the phone. She is well spoken and direct, and hardly needs me to convey her words.

So, the following is what she wrote to me:

I had an idyllic childhood. Although I was born in England, my father was an officer in the British Army so we lived abroad during my formative years – in Germany and North Africa. I have vivid memories of school in the morning and then down to the beach in the afternoon, amazing sandstorms, a veranda around the house filled with red geraniums and the evocative smells of an African country.

My secondary education was spent at a boarding school which I loathed. Thankfully my parents allowed me to do my A levels at a sixth form college in Winchester, which is where we have always had a home – rather like a bolt-hole to which we could return after foreign postings.

I then joined the army myself – no real connection to my father's profession. I turned down my place at university; I had itchy feet and needed a change. So I had eight years of great fun and, in my last posting, where I worked closely with an advertising agency, I had more business lunches per week than my husband did!

My next move was into sports car racing where I helped run the World Championship and travelled to various places. Le Mans was fantastic fun but quite stressful as one had to remain awake and alert for over twenty-four hours – dealing with team problems, meeting drivers and keeping race officials happy. Can I blame my cancer on a liquid diet of coffee and endless croque monsieurs? I think not.

I remember little about my diet during my childhood except that my mother was a good cook. We drank full-fat milk, ate butter and quite a lot of meat. Pasta was not as popular as it is today but there were, luckily, very few convenience foods. There was always fruit available and I feel our diet was pretty well balanced.

In 1982 I met and married my husband Rupert who worked in the City. Five years after, Harriet was born, and two years later her brother, Edward. Life was great.

But then the bubble burst. It was Rupert who first noticed the lump, in May 1995. It was about the size of a cherry. I went to the doctor immediately and was slightly disconcerted when she recommended it be checked out further. An appointment was made for three months later – *three months*! I just simply couldn't believe that I was expected to wait that length of time and so decided to go private. I was seen two days later and it seemed that the lump was some sort of cyst but would need removing. I went into hospital a week later.

I awoke from the surgery to hear Rupert and the consultant talking outside the room. Suddenly I had the most awful sinking feeling and I knew I had cancer. When the surgeon came in to see me, he said that he had done a lumpectomy as cancerous cells had been found in the tumour. I was unable to say anything as I was so full of morphine and remained completely out of it for the rest of the day.

The next day dawned, and when I woke up and saw Rupert beside me, I just cried. I did not want to die. To me, cancer meant only one thing – death. When I left hospital I had to tell the family, which was not easy. Trying to explain to children something like that is incredibly hard. My five year-old son asked me if I was going to die. When I told him that I hoped not, he replied, 'That's okay then!' and ran off outside to play football. My daughter was extremely concerned and needed to be told everything. I felt that I should be totally honest with them and I do believe it worked. They were able to cope with all the hospital visits, the treatment and all my mood swings because they knew (God, how I hoped it was the truth) that I was not going to die but that I would be unwell at times until I got better.

I decided to tell everyonc and this policy was good for me. People were very kind and no one ever crossed the road to avoid me! My parents and sister were fantastic and friends were wonderful. Rupert was amazing, and even though I rarely cried he always listened to me, even when I must have sounded like a stuck record.

My prognosis was good – the tumour had been caught early. But as a preventative measure, I was to have a course of radiotherapy and chemotherapy. However, before all the treatment started I had various tests which included a bone scan. The results of this showed a 'hot spot' of activity in my jaw. So, two weeks after the first operation, I was back under anaesthetic to investigate this.

With a bit of my jaw removed, I went back to work. Then a couple of days later I went to be measured up for my radiotherapy. While I was there, the radiologist examined me, felt under my arms and then said that I must see my oncologist immediately. I walked out of the room and had my first and only panic attack. I assumed from this meeting that he had discovered more cancer and I really couldn't cope with it.

Two weeks later I was back in hospital yet again, this time to have some lymph nodes removed. This was the worst of all the operations as the recovery period was so painful and I was in hospital for much longer than before. Fortunately the results were good – there was no cancer spread to the glands and the results of the previous operation to my jaw were also negative.

After this came the radiotherapy, everyday for six weeks. I had some counselling at this point because I felt poor Rupert was getting bored with hearing about all my guilt. It was a real luxury to sit in a stranger's office and cry for a whole hour once a week! I stopped these sessions when I felt that even the counsellor must be getting bored with hearing the same things each week!

Once the summer was over, the chemotherapy loomed. I felt tired from the radiotherapy but well. It was horrible to go deliberately and be injected with poisons and be made to feel unwell. I was on a three-week cycle: two weeks feeling great, a blood test and chemo and then a week feeling rough, and it continued like that for nearly six months. Fortunately I had some fantastic anti-sickness pills and my hair didn't fall out. However I did hate those injections.

Nearly a year later and I was told that I needed no further treatment other than Tamoxifen, and periodic check-ups. Nearly four years later, and I'm feeling very well and back to full energy levels. I have started my own nursery school, which is exciting, and which I hope will be successful. My own children seem to be unscarred by this experience and appear to be as before – growing like weeds and enjoying life!

I wish I could say I was a better person as a result of my trauma but I can't. I have rather a short fuse now and get cross or upset much more easily than I did before. I salve my conscience by helping various breast cancer charities as much as I can.

Some time ago I had a severe pain in my ribs. I had it checked out at the local breast clinic but they didn't know what it was. In fact I had a fractured rib! Now I've been told it is a side effect of the radiotherapy to have a brittle rib. A small price to pay for my life!

Julia's Sister Deborah's Story

We had been trying to convince ourselves that Julia's breast lump was nothing to worry about. But then she phoned to tell me that it was malignant. She was very calm. She'd done her crying with Rupert. I'm not sure what I said, so many thoughts were rushing through my head. What about Harriet and Edward? Would she die? I wouldn't be able to phone her up and have a good moan. What about treatment? Was she getting the best care? And of course, that horrible stomach-churning thought – would I get it too?

I then went into overdrive, phoning medical friends for information, finding out if Julia's consultant had a good reputation. The desire to help was overpowering; I wanted to do as much as I could for Julia. Harriet and Edward came to stay while she had the operations, I visited Julia in hospital and even accompanied her when she had the radiotherapy and Rupert couldn't get the time off.

I talked to Rupert to make sure he was okay because he was being drained by all the worry. I was also aware of how awful the situation was for my parents – their daughter had breast cancer. They did not live nearby and therefore couldn't help out as much as they wanted to. We all spent ages on the telephone supporting each other.

It's now nearly four years on and Julia looks wonderful and is full of energy. We spend a lot of time together but the worry of the cancer is always at the back of our minds.

Chapter XII
Doreen Hinder

Doreen Hinder lives in Stanwix, Carlisle with her husband. Her breast cancer was diagnosed in 1996 while in her fifties. She underwent a mastectomy and was put on Tamoxifen. She has since had reconstructive surgery.

Doreen's Story

The first letter I received from Doreen was a very short, polite letter, but her sincerity shone through, and the last sentence read, 'If my simple story is of help, I will be more than happy to supply more details.' Although, at this moment of writing, I have not met Doreen, from our communication so far I feel that the genuine, caring personality that I have formulated in my own head is not wrong.

She was born in 1938 in Rochford, just outside Southend-on-Sea in Essex. Her parents had married late in life and her mother was forty-one when she had Doreen and there was already an older brother.

Her father had farmed in Canada for many years before, but when the Depression came he returned to England, only to encounter the Depression here. He took casual work and didn't get regular work until the Second World War. Consequently, the family was quite poor. They lived in a council house in Southend until all women and children were evacuated. Doreen, her mother and brother went to live with relatives in Devon and stayed there until she was four.

She says that they were quite lucky as far as diet went. There were never any times of hunger, at least not that she can remember. There was always plenty of milk and vegetables and they had a monthly food parcel sent from relatives in Canada.

After they had returned to Southend, Doreen went to the local primary school and then won a scholarship to go to Ackworth, a Quaker boarding school in Yorkshire. She describes the diet here as wholesome! To a child it would have seemed very plain and bland – wholemeal bread, meat and vegetables, sweets only playing a small part.

She had little idea of what she wanted to do after school, and as she was sports mad, decided to join the WRAF when she was seventeen and a half. She worked as an operations clerk at several different bases throughout the UK. During these four years, she felt some kind of religious calling, and after leaving the WRAF, went to Selly Oak to train as a deaconess. She later became a Baptist minister.

In 1978, she married her husband Geoff. She had met him when she became the minister of the church he attended down in Somerset. In 1980 they moved to Scotland with Geoff's work and then in 1986 to Carlisle, which is where they still live today.

The cancer problem started in 1995. It was the week between Christmas and the new year. She was taking a shower and noticed something different about her left breast. There wasn't a lump, more like a thickening. She regularly checked herself and it was probably because of this that she detected the slight change. She felt scared and unsure. She didn't know whether something was wrong or not so decided to see the local practice nurse for a second opinion. However, there weren't many people around so was sent to see the duty doctor. He examined her and said he thought there was nothing wrong but to put Doreen's mind at rest, would arrange for her to go to the hospital.

Very much relieved, she put the experience to the back of her mind. She went to see the consultant on 7th February 1996. She had a mammogram and an ultrasound scan and she remembers the operator who was doing the test telling her it was probably a case of mastitis. Again she took comfort from these remarks. However, two days later the hospital sent for her to go in again and this time the consultant carried out a needle biopsy. Thankfully Geoff was with her on this occasion as she was feeling very nervous and the consultant made no mention of mastitis.

On 15th February, a MacMillan nurse called and said that she needed to have a biopsy done the following day. Geoff took her to hospital on the sixteenth. They both felt very anxious. When she saw the consultant he told her that they had found a few suspect cells and that was the reason for the biopsy.

When the nurse phoned her on the twentieth asking Doreen to see the consultant the next day, she knew it was bad news. But even when he did actually tell her that she had a cancerous tumour, it still came as a shock. She was asked whether she wanted a mastectomy or a lumpectomy which she found very difficult to answer, partly because she felt so confused trying to absorb everything, and also because she had no knowledge that could help her make the best decision. In the end, she opted for a mastectomy and implant, based on the assumption that if she got rid of as much tissue as possible, she would then stand a better chance of survival. This actually proved to be the right choice in the end, because during her operation, cancer cells were found throughout the breast and not just localised to the tumour site.

The next few days were harrowing. Doreen rang family and friends who offered support. She and Geoff talked a lot, and although they were both very emotional, they also kept a very positive attitude. On the twenty-third, they went to the hospital for Doreen to be measured for the reconstruction. She was also given some pamphlets about breast cancer to read. That Sunday, the congregation at her church prayed for her well-being, which Doreen herself says she found very supportive and comforting.

And so the day came. Geoff drove her to the hospital on the twenty-eighth. She had a side room on the ward which she had chosen so that she could be alone. The mastectomy was done the following day, and for the next couple of days Doreen felt very sick, probably from the anaesthetic. Not long after, she started to feel much better and her appetite returned. But then suddenly, six days after her operation, she burst into tears. Reality hit home as she confronted life after losing her breast, and the fears that her husband might no longer love her were mounting. She was comforted by the staff and found them very kind and supportive. Later that evening, the consultant visited her with good news this time. The lymph glands were clear and this would greatly enhance her survival. Geoff and Doreen just cried with relief – their happiness was immense. She finally went home on 15th March, just over two weeks after her surgery.

No further treatment was necessary other than taking Tamoxifen, and Doreen has since had the reconstruction done.

Doreen feels that stress was a key factor in triggering her cancer. There was no history of breast cancer in her family before and she herself admits that she has a high-achieving personality.

But some good has come out of this experience for her. It has given her a sense of joy for life and living. She says that being aware of your own mortality and having to come to terms with the thought of death is very hard and makes a person very fearful, but for her, now, those fears have passed and she is now able to get on with life. She feels that each day is a gift, one that she is grateful for beyond doubt!

Doreen's Husband Geoff's Story

At first, when Doreen told me of the strange feeling in her breast, the thought of cancer never entered my head. I accompanied Doreen whenever she had to go to hospital, not only to support her, but also to be with her if she should be told bad news. When eventually we were told that she had breast cancer, my initial thought was that this sort of thing only happened to other people. Once it had sunk in, I just felt that I wanted to support Doreen and to help beat this illness together.

The decision to have the mastectomy instead of a lumpectomy was a joint one. I didn't mind what Doreen's physical appearance would be afterwards, I just wanted to make a choice that would help her survival. During the days leading up to her operation, we continued to live a normal life, and carried out all our usual commitments. I was not willing to let the situation get on top of us.

The most anxious time was waiting to see if the disease had spread. When the consultant told us that the cancer had been confined to the breast I burst into tears. It had obviously been an emotional strain, and the relief was immense.

I am very proud of Doreen – she is a very courageous lass. My love for her is as strong as ever and I am glad she is able to support the local Breast Cancer Support Group which means so much to her.

Chapter XIII
Sylvia Richards-Jones, MBE

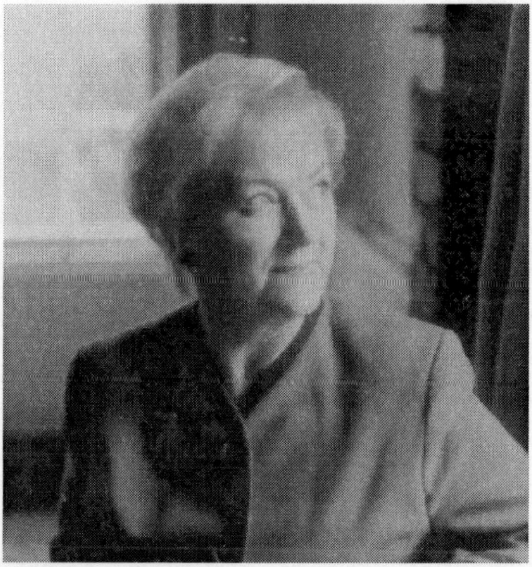

Photo by Clare Shvili, 1998

Sylvia Richards-Jones, MBE lives in Brymbo, Wrexham with her husband. They have two grown-up children and two grandchildren. She was diagnosed in 1996 when in her late fifties. After having a mastectomy, she was put on Tamoxifen.

Sylvia's Story

Looking at the photograph that Sylvia sent to me, it's hard to imagine that she's had breast cancer. She's a very attractive woman, and, judging by her appearance, obviously takes great care with the way she looks. On the telephone she comes across as the sort of person who knows exactly what she likes and what she doesn't! She's direct and confident, which I suppose isn't very surprising for an ex-headteacher.

She is the last contributor to this book, but certainly by no means the least. She has been successful in life, as her MBE would suggest, and of course, she has come out the other side of a bad experience shining.

Sylvia was born in Wrexham in 1937 of Welsh parents. She was educated at Grove Park Grammar School for Girls in Wrexham. Her first job was as a nursery nurse at a local infant school. In 1963 she qualified as a teacher of special needs children at a college in Manchester. She taught at two special needs schools up until she got the post of headteacher at a school in Flintshire in 1971. At that time, she was the youngest headteacher in the county. In 1984 she was awarded the MBE for her services to Education, having been headteacher at three Flintshire schools. She is now in retirement.

Sylvia is married to Terry, who is a retired BT engineer. They have a daughter, Alison, who in 1988 gained her BSc degree in Physiotherapy and is married with two children. They also have a son, Neil, who graduated in 1993 having attained a BN honours degree and who lives in Macclesfield with his girlfriend.

Her story starts in March 1996, when Sylvia was informed by Flintshire County Council that her request for early retirement had been accepted and that the date was confirmed as 31st August of that year. In fact the retirement date would coincide with the silver anniversary of her becoming a headteacher, which seemed very appropriate.

In April 1996, she contacted the practice nurse at her local surgery to ask how she could get a mammogram done, as for the previous couple of months she had been aware that her right breast was quite painful. Although at first she put it down to normal monthly tenderness, when it got worse her husband suggested she should see the GP.

The nurse made an appointment for Sylvia to see the doctor. Two days later she saw him about the pain and discomfort and pointed out that her next routine mammogram wasn't until the end of 1996. He examined her and said there weren't any signs of a lump but he was quite happy to make a referral, and promptly. He also said that having pain in the breast was very rarely a sign of something sinister. This is in fact true, but of course she was still worried, even though only slightly. She went for the mammogram then carried on as normal, even offering reassurance to people who were concerned for her!

But then in the Easter holidays while she was at home, she received a call from the GP asking her to go and see him urgently. He told her that a shadow had shown up on the x-ray and that he was going to refer her to see a consultant at Wrexham Hospital.

On 23rd April she saw the consultant. He too could find no evidence of a lump but wanted Sylvia to go into hospital to have a biopsy done. It was 6th May when she went in, and by now she had noticed for the first time a slight puckering of skin on her breast. Ten days later she and her husband went back to the hospital for the results. The surgeon who had operated confirmed that she had breast cancer. They both just broke down, and her immediate thought was that she wouldn't see her grandchildren grow up. She asked if she could phone her daughter with the news, who went straightaway to be with her parents and listen to what the surgeon said. He told them that there were two options open to Sylvia, either to have a lumpectomy followed by radiotherapy, or to have a mastectomy and decide about any necessary treatment at a later date once the cancer had been graded. Without hesitation, she decided to have a mastectomy.

On 5th June, Sylvia went into hospital once again. She had thought about the consequences of a mastectomy long and hard, and felt that losing a breast would not affect her sexuality. That was one thing she was very confident about. And her husband Terry was very supportive, saying that he had married her for the person she was and quipped afterwards that he was a 'legs' man anyway!

Following the surgery, Sylvia only needed very small amounts of pain relief and was very surprised at the lack of pain she felt. Before she left hospital on 14th June, the consultant visited her with all the results from the operation. He told her they had found three tumours in all, two deep in the breast and one in a lymph gland, and that the histology report showed that the cancer had been there for approximately eight to twelve months. Fortunately, the grade was low and no further treatment was necessary apart from taking Tamoxifen. As she left hospital, she still had one of the drains left intact because of complications. She had to keep the drain in for nine long weeks after, during which time one of the local community nurses visited on a daily basis to check it. Sylvia also went to the hospital every week until eventually the drain was taken out.

The first outpatient appointment was in July and she was then prescribed Tamoxifen, having been told about the possible side effects and the benefits.

Almost three years later, she still has her hospital check-ups which have been extended to every nine months. The only problem has been with lymphodema which she developed in her right arm and part of her trunk area. She has received water therapy treatment and physiotherapy at a local hospice to try and help the problem.

When she first had to go to the hospice, her initial reaction was anxiety at being sent to a place that she had always associated with terminally ill patients. But after seeing what really goes on inside the hospice, she has changed her mind and now looks forward to her visits because of the positive approach shown by all the staff, and of course the love and friendship that the patients receive.

Before and after her surgery, Sylvia was visited by a breast care nurse who was able to advise about the practicalities of having a mastectomy. She was also able to offer Sylvia support and counselling, which has been of great value. This was highlighted at one point when Sylvia was very afraid that because of the lymph gland involvement, she was going to die. Two days later when the breast care nurse came to see her, she explained the laboratory findings in great depth and put Sylvia's mind at rest. She now feels very strongly that every breast cancer patient should be linked up with such a nurse.

She is now very positive and says her philosophy now is 'Don't spend time worrying about things that you have no control over concentrate on what you can change!' She has been reminded about how precious and exciting life really is.

As a family, although they have always been close, the ordeal has made them even closer and stronger. But one concern Sylvia does have is for all families who experience breast cancer and the emotions they have to go through alone. She remembers thinking how stressed her husband looked the day after her mastectomy, probably more so than she actually was.

She feels very lucky to have such good friends who have given her the strength she needed. And her circle of friends is growing through her committee work for the charity

Breakthrough. She and Terry are enjoying a 'quality' retirement together and this year, they celebrate their Ruby Wedding anniversary. They have joined a fitness club and she has even learnt to swim after thirty years of trying!

The final word goes to Sylvia:

> It is important to try and not make yourself a victim of disease: life is for living. And yes, believe me, there is a quality of life after breast cancer, provided you are prepared to make it happen. I have!

Sylvia's Daughter Alison's Story

Initially, when Mum went for the mammogram, I was not concerned at all, and even when she was asked to see the GP I was still not terribly troubled by this. Mum was however somewhat nervous and I did my best to reassure her that there was nothing to worry about.

Then I went with her for the first appointment with the consultant. After, she was upset that she hadn't been given any kind of indication about whether there was something serious or not, and although I had started to suspect it could be cancer, I tried to be positive, both for her and myself.

The day of the biopsy was a difficult one for us all. I was concerned in case she had a frozen section done and then had to have a mastectomy. I couldn't concentrate on work, and eventually rang the ward to see how she was and what had been done. The nurse said he wasn't allowed to discuss anything over the telephone but would speak to me if I went in. Now I was convinced of the worst. By the time I reached the hospital, I was almost in tears, but when I got to the ward, there was Mum, sitting up in bed with her lipstick on and fingernails painted! I cannot describe how relieved I was.

Waiting for the results was unbearable. On the day, I was at home with my husband and children. I can honestly say it was the worst day of my life. Then Mum phoned with the news, and after putting the phone down, I just cried and cried. I went straight to the hospital to be with Mum and Dad and we all cried together.

After the mastectomy had been done, we were told that Mum didn't need any further treatment, and I began to relax more. Before this I had frequently cried myself to sleep, wondering how much longer Mum would be around.

The whole experience has changed my view about breast cancer, and although I am aware of the slightly increased risk of my developing the disease, I am not overly concerned. It has highlighted my family's mortality and now makes me appreciate them more than ever.

Advisory Services

BREAKTHROUGH
Kingsway House
Kingsway
London WC2
Telephone: 0171 405 511

CANCERLINK
11–21 Northdown Street
London N1 9BN
Information: 0800 132 905
Asian Line: 0800 590 415
Young People: 0800 591 028
(Freephone helplines)

BACUP (British Association of Cancer United Patients)
3 Bath Place
London EC2
Cancer Information Centre Linkline: 0800 181 199
Counselling: 0171 696 9000

BREAST CANCER CARE
Anchor House
15 Britten Street
London SW3
Telephone: 0171 867 9303
Helpline: 0171 384 2344
Nationwide Freeline Freecall: 0500 245 345